I of the Vortex

From Neurons to Self

Rodolfo R. Llinás

A Bradford Book
The MIT Press
Cambridge, Massachusetts
London, England

This book was set in Sabon and Meta by Wellington Graphics, Westwood, Massachusetts.

Printed and bound in the United States of America.

Library of Congress Cataloging-in-Publication Data

Llinás, Rodolfo R. (Rodolfo Riascos), 1934–
  I of the vortex : from neurons to self / Rodolfo Llinás.
    p. cm.
  "A Bradford book."
  Includes bibliographical references and index.
  ISBN 0-262-12233-2 (alk. paper)
    1. Consciousness. 2. Brain. 3. Neural networks (Neurobiology) 4. Brain—Evolution. I. Title.

QP411 .L56 2000
612.8′2—dc21   00-041863

Contents

Preface

This essay arose out of a set of talks given at The University of St. Andrews in Scotland, where Professor Glen Cottrell had graciously invited me to give the American Alumni Lectures in 1989. Little did I know then that St. Andrews would be back in my life, when, in 1998, my son Alexander obtained his Ph.D. there during a break in his medical studies at New York University.

The generation of this essay owes much to Michael Kistler, to whom I dictated much of this manuscript, so giving me a leg up into getting the material into a form that I could work with. Dr. Jean Jacoby helped with the editing. My son Rafael, presently a junior staff neurologist at Harvard's Beth Israel Hospital, took the time to read and criticize this effort, as did my wife, Dr. Gillian Kimber, from her perspective as a philosopher of mind. I would also like to thank a special friend, Dr. Antonio Fernandez de Molina, and my colleague Dr. Kerry Walton for special comments and additions.

This book presents a personal view of neuroscience aimed toward a general audience, as well as toward students and those of my colleagues who might enjoy an attempt at synthesis. This general view is offered from the perspective of a single-cell physiologist interested in neuronal integration and synaptic transmission. Such a position is privileged, because it lies between the realms of the molecular and the systemic, as they relate to brain function.

Single large neurons have physical dimensions observable at low optimal magnification, that of a tenth of a millimeter. That is big enough to be dissected by hand with pins, using a good magnifying glass (Deiters 1856). Moving just two orders of magnitude down to the micrometer level, which requires a good microscope, one is at the scale of synaptic transmission. One may observe synapses at the union between nerve and muscle, for example. Two orders of magnitude further down, at tens of nanometers, with the aid of electron microscopy, we find the realm of single ion channels and of signal transduction and molecular biology.

If, on the other hand we wish to roam orders of magnitude above the physiology of single cells, we find at two orders of magnitude above, and in the centimeter realm, the world of systems that is the scale of pennies, buttons, and fingernails. At a further two orders of magnitude up, we come to meters and to the world of motricity and cognition that characterizes human beings. That is, we arrive at the realm of chairs and telephones and other objects that one can hold in one's hand or under one's arm.

Most neuroscientists feel that two orders of magnitude above and below one's central focus is "horizon enough," and that anyone attempting four orders above and below is reckless. However, there are some who attempt such a dangerous dynamic range. They probably know that the risk of failure is the price of synthesis, without which there are only fields of dismembered parts.

Motor Primacy and the Organization of Neuronal Networks: Thinking as Internalized Movement

A fundamental first step in exploring the nature of mind, from a scientific point of view, is to reject the premise that the mind appeared suddenly as a result of spectacular intervention. The nature of mind must be understood on the basis of its origin, the process of its becoming, by the biological mechanism of trial and error endlessly at work. The mind, or what I shall refer to as the "mindness state," is the product of evolutionary processes that have occurred in the brain as actively moving creatures developed from the primitive to the highly evolved. Therefore, a true examination of the scientific basis for mindness requires a rigorous evolutionary perspective, as it is through this process that mindness came to be. How the mind came to us (or we to it, as we shall see) is a rich and beautiful story that is over 700 million years old—and, like all things biological, is still being written.

A prerequisite for grasping the nature of mind is, first and foremost, the appropriate perspective. Just as Western society, steeped in dualistic thinking, must re-orient in order to grasp the elemental tenets of nondualistic philosophy, so there must be a fundamental reorientation of perspective in order to approach the neurobiological nature of mind. An attempt at such reorienting was the task in the American Alumni Lectures at St. Andrews; this book will proceed in that vein.

Charles Sherrington, in his Gifford Lectures at Edinburgh in 1937, entitled *Man on his Nature* (1941, chapter 12), hinted at the possibility that if human beings ever came face to face with their true natures that knowledge might trigger the demise of human civilization. To him, evidently, humans prefer to consider themselves the lowest of angels rather than the highest of beasts. I am of the opinion that if we were to comprehend fully the awesome nature of mindness, we would, in fact, respect and admire each other all the more.

I of the Vortex

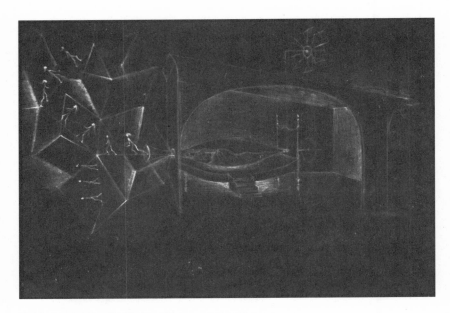

R. Vario, *Sueño*, 1958. Pencil/paper, 23 × 16 cm.

1

Setting Mind to Mind

Mindness, Global Function Brain States, and Sensorimotor Images

There are some basic guidelines to be considered when taking a scientific approach to the mind. Because this book is not supposed to be a detective story, let me offer some demarcating/clarifying definitions of the mind or "mindness state" that will be used here. From my monist's perspective, the brain and the mind are inseparable events. Moreover, the mind, or mindness state, is but one of several global functional states generated by the brain. Mind or the mindness state, is that class of all functional brain states in which sensorimotor images, including self-awareness, are generated. When using the term sensorimotor image, I mean something more than visual imagery. I refer to the conjunction or binding of all relevant sensory input to produce a discreet functional state that ultimately may result in action. For instance, imagine that you have an itch on your back, at a place that you cannot see but which generates an internal "image" giving you a location within the complex geography of your body as well as an attitude to take: SCRATCH! That is a sensorimotor image. The generation of a sensorimotor image is not a simple input/output response, or a reflex, because it occurs within the context of what the animal is presently doing. For obvious reasons, a dog wouldn't want to scratch with one leg while another one is up in the air. So, context is as important as content in the generation of sensorimotor images and premotor formulation.

There are other states that occupy the same space in the brain mass but which may not support awareness. These include being asleep, being drugged or anesthetized, or having a grand mal epileptic seizure. When one's brain is in these states, consciousness is lost; all memories and feelings melt into nothingness; yet the brain continues to function, requiring its normal supply of oxygen and nutrients. During these states, the brain does not generate awareness of any kind, not even of one's own existence (self-awareness). It does not generate our worries, our hopes, or our fears—all is oblivion.

By contrast, I consider the global brain state known as dreaming to be a cognitive state, but not with respect to co-existing external reality because it is not directly modulated by one's senses (Llinás & Pare 1991). Rather, this state draws from the past experiences stored in our brain or from the intrinsic workings of the brain itself. Yet another global brain state would be that known as "lucid dreaming" (LaBerge & Rheingold 1990), where one is actually aware that one is dreaming.

In short then, the brain is more than the one and a half liters of inert grayish matter occasionally seen pickled in a jar atop some dusty laboratory shelf. One should think of the brain as a living entity that generates well-defined electrical activity. This activity could be described perhaps as "self-controlled" electrical storms, or what Charles Sherrington (1941, p. 225), one of the pioneers of neuroscience, refers to as the "enchanted loom." In the wider context of neuronal networks, this activity is the mind.

This mind is co-dimensional with the brain; it occupies all of the brain's nooks and crannies. But as with an electrical storm, the mind does not represent at any given time all possible storms, only those isomorphic with (re-enacting, a transformed recreation of) *the state of the local surrounding world as we observe it* when we are awake. When dreaming, as we are released from the tyranny of our sensory input, the system generates intrinsic storms that create "possible" worlds—perhaps—very much as we do when we think.

Living brains and their electrical storms are descriptors for different aspects of the same thing, namely neuronal function. These days, one hears metaphors for central nervous system function that are derived from the world of computers, such as "the brain is hardware and the mind, software" (see discussion by Block 1995). I think this type of language usage is totally misleading. In the working brain, the "hardware" and the "software" are intertwined in the functional units, the neurons themselves. Neurons are both "the early bird" *and* "the worm," because mindness coincides with functional brain states.

Before returning to our discussion of mindness, think about the itch on your back again, and in particular the moment of the sensorimotor image—before you put into action the motor event of scratching the itch. Can you recognize the sense of future inherent to sensorimotor images, the pulling toward the action to be performed? This is very important, and a very old part of mindness. From the earliest dawning of biological evolution it was this governing, this leading, this pulling by predictive drive, *intention,* that brought sensorimotor images—indeed, the mind itself—to us in the first place.

Let us shore up the discussion with a bit more precision. I propose that this mindness state, which may or may not represent external reality (the latter as with imagining or dreaming), has evolved as a goal-oriented device that implements predictive/intentional interactions between a living organism and its environment. Such transactions, to be successful, require an inherited, prewired instrument that generates an internal image of the external world that can then be compared with sensory-transduced information from the external environment. All of this must be supported in real time. The functional comparison of internally generated sensorimotor images with real-time sensory information from an organism's immediate environment is known as perception. Underlying the workings of perception is prediction, that is, the useful expectation of events yet to come. Prediction, with its goal-oriented essence, so very different from reflex, is the very core of brain function.

Why Is Mindness So Mysterious?

Why is mindness so mysterious to us? Why has it always been this way? The processes that generate such states as thinking, consciousness, and dreaming are foreign to us, I fancy, because they always seem to be generated with no apparent relation to the external world. They seem impalpably internal.

At New York University School of Medicine, in a lecture in honor of the late Professor Homer Smith, entitled, "Unity of Organic Design: From Goethe and Geoffrey Chaucer to Homology of Homeotic Complexes in Anthropods and Vertebrates," Stephen J. Gould mentioned the well-known evolutionary hypothesis that we vertebrates may be regarded as crustaceans turned inside out. We are endoskeletal, with an internal skeleton; crustaceans are exoskeletal, with an external skeleton.

This idea led me to consider what would have happened if we had remained exoskeletal? If we had an external skeleton, the concept of how movement is generated might be just as incomprehensible to us as is the concept of thinking or mindness. Having an internal skeleton means that we become quite aware of our muscles from birth. We can see their movement and feel their contractions and clearly understand, in a very intimate way, their relation to the movement of our different body parts. Unfortunately, we do not have such direct knowledge concerning the workings of our brain. Why not? Because from a cerebral mass point of view, we are crustaceans—our brains and spinal cord are covered by exoskeleton! (figure 1.1).

If we could observe or feel the brain at work, it would be immediately obvious that neuronal function is as related to how we see, interpret, and react, as muscle contractions are related to the movements we make. As for our crustacean friends, who lack the luxury of direct knowledge of the relationship of muscle contraction to movement, their movement ability, if they could consider it, *might* seem as inexplicable to them as thinking or mindness is to us. The essential point is that we do understand about muscles and tendons; in fact, we revel in them. We go so far as to hold world competitions for the comparison of symmetrically hypertrophied muscle mass produced by obsessively "pumping iron" (and occasionally popping steroids), even though, as physical strength for size

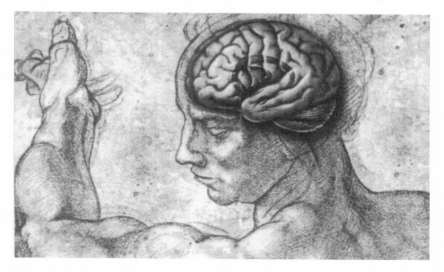

Figure 1.1
Detail showing the upper body and head from a life drawing by Leonardo da Vinci, with an image of the brain superimposed.

goes in the animal kingdom, we are way down near the bottom of the heap. The more analytically probing among us employ measuring tapes, scales, and force transducers in an effort to describe the properties of these precious organs of movement. However, no such paraphernalia are available for directly assessing the working of the brain (IQ tests not withstanding). Perhaps this is why, in the field of neuroscience, such differing concepts have arisen about how the brain is functionally organized.

The central generation of movement and the generation of mindness are deeply related; they are in fact different parts of the same process. In my view, from its very evolutionary inception mindness is the internalization of movement.

Historical Views of Motor Organization in the Brain

Around the turn of this century, there arose two strong opposing views on the subject of the execution of movement. The first, championed by

William James (1890), viewed the working organization of the central nervous system as fundamentally reflexological. From this perspective the brain is essentially a complex input/output system driven by the momentary demands of the environment. Production of movement must be driven by sensation, and the generation of movement is fundamentally a response to a sensory cue. This basic idea was very influential in the groundbreaking studies of Charles Sherrington and his school (1948). It provided the impetus for the study of central reflexes—their function and how they were organized—and ultimately for the study of central synaptic transmission and neuronal integration. All of these have played crucial roles in present-day neuroscience.

A second influential approach was championed by Graham Brown (1911, 1914, 1915). Brown believed that the spinal cord was not organized reflexologically. He viewed this system as organized on a self-referential basis by central neuronal circuits that provided the drive for the electrical pattern generation required for organized movement. This conclusion was based on his studies of locomotion in deafferented animals, that is, animals in which the pathways bringing sensation from the legs to the spinal cord are severed. Under these conditions animals could still produce an organized gait (Brown 1911). This led Brown to propose that movement, even organized movement, is intrinsically generated in the absence of sensory input. He viewed reflex activity as required only for the modulation of, rather than being the driving force for, the production of gait. So, for example, while locomotion (one step after the other) is organized intrinsically, not requiring input from the external world, sensory input (e.g., a slippery spot on the ground) reflexively resets the rhythm so that we don't fall, but it does not generate walking itself.

Brown went on to propose that locomotion is produced in the spinal cord by reciprocal neuronal activity. In very simplified terms, autonomous neuronal networks on one side of the spinal cord activate the muscles of the limb on the same side while preventing activity by the opposite limb. He described this reciprocal organization as "half-paired centers" (Brown 1914), as their mutual interaction generated the left/right limb pacing that is locomotion (see figure 2.5, below).

In this context, the function of the sensory input giving rise to reflex activity during locomotion is there to modulate the ongoing activity of the spinal cord motor network in order to adapt the activity (the output signal) to the irregularities of the terrain over which the animal moves. We now know that such ongoing activity born of the intrinsic electrical activity of neurons in the spinal cord and brain stem forms the basis for both breathing (Feldman et al. 1990) and locomotion (Stein et al. 1986; Cohen 1987; Grillner and Matsushima 1991; Lansner et al. 1998) in vertebrates. A similar dynamic organization, but supported by a quite different anatomical arrangement, is found in invertebrates (Marder 1998). In both vertebrates and invertebrates, the neuronal activity being transmitted and modified between different levels by synaptic connectivity has comparable dynamic properties.

Brown's views remain highly regarded by many of us and have been seminal to our understanding of the intrinsic activity of central neurons (Llinás 1974, 1988; Stein et al. 1984). This conceptual view of spinal cord function may be extended to the workings of the brainstem and areas of higher brain function, such as the thalamus and forebrain—areas where mindness is ultimately generated in our brain.

The Intrinsic Nature of Brain Function

A working hypothesis related to Brown's ideas is that nervous system function may actually operate on its own, intrinsically, and that sensory input modulates rather than informs this intrinsic system (Llinás 1974). Let me hasten to say that being disconnected from sensory input is *not* the normal operational mode of the brain, as we all know from childhood, when first we observed the behavior of a deaf or blind person. But the exact opposite is equally untrue: the brain does not depend on continuous input from the external world to generate perceptions (see *The Last Hippie,* by Oliver Sacks), but only to modulate them contextually. If one accepts this view, it follows that the brain, like the heart, operates as a self-referential, closed system in at least two different senses: one, as something separated from our direct inquiry by implacable bone; and two, as a system that is mostly self-referential, only able to know universals by means of specialized sense organs. Evolution suggests that these sense organs specify internal states that reflect neuronal circuit selection derived from ancestral trial and error. Such circuits become genetically predetermined (for example, we can see color primarily without having to learn to do so). Once we are born, these ancestral circuits (comprising the inherited, functional architecture of the brain) are further enriched by our own experiences as individuals and thus constitute our own particular memories, indeed, our selves.

We can look to the world of neurology for support of the concept that the brain operates as a closed system, a system in which the role of sensory input appears to be weighted more toward the specification of ongoing cognitive states than toward the supply of information—context over content. This is no different than sensory input modulating a pattern of neural activity generated in the spinal cord to produce walking, except that here we are talking of a cognitive state generated by the brain and how sensory input modulates such a state. The principle is the same. For example, prosopagnosia is a condition in which individuals, due to neurological damage, cannot recognize human faces. They can see and recognize the different parts of a face, as well as subtle facial features, but not the face as a whole entity (Damasio et al. 1982; De Renzi and Pellegrino, 1998). Moreover, the people that inhabit the dreams of prosopagnostics are faceless (Llinás and Pare 1991) (we shall return to this issue later in the book).

The significance of sensory cues is expressed mainly by their incorporation into larger, cognitive states or entities. In other words, sensory cues earn representation via their impact upon the pre-existing functional disposition of the brain (Llinás 1974, 1987). This concept, that the significance of incoming sensory information depends on the pre-existing functional disposition of the brain, is a far deeper issue than one gathers at first glance—particularly when we look into questions of the nature of "self."

Intrinsic Electrical Properties of Neurons: Oscillation, Resonance, Rhythmicity, and Coherence

How, then, do central neurons organize and drive bodily movement, create sensorimotor images, and generate our thoughts? Having grown in our knowledge from the days of Brown, we may paraphrase the above question today to read: How do the intrinsic oscillatory properties of central neurons relate to the information-carrying properties of the brain as a whole? Before attempting to answer this question, there are still a few more terms to cover. Let me start by describing what is meant by the intrinsic oscillatory electrical properties of the brain, from a relatively nontechnical point of view. This concept is at the heart of all we shall discuss in this book.

Oscillation

When one thinks of the word "oscillation," one thinks of a rhythmic back-and-forth event. Pendulums oscillate, as do metronomes; they are periodic oscillators. The sweeping motion of a lamprey's tail, back and forth, as it swims (Cohen 1987; Grillner and Matsushima 1991) is a wonderful example of an oscillatory movement.

Many of the types of neurons in the nervous system are endowed with particular types of intrinsic electrical activity that imbue them with particular functional properties. Such electrical activity is manifested as variations in the minute voltage across the cell's enveloping membrane (Llinás 1988). This voltage may oscillate in a manner similar to the traveling, sinusoidal waves that we see as gentle ripples in calm water, and are weakly chaotic (Makarenko and Llinás 1998). As we will see later, this confers a great temporal agility to the system. These oscillations of voltage remain in the local vicinity of the neuron's body and dendrites, and have frequencies ranging from less than one per second to more than forty per second. On these voltage ripples, and in particular on their crests, much larger electrical events known as action potentials may be evoked; these are powerful and far reaching electrical signals that form the basis for neuron-to-neuron communication. Action potentials are the messages that travel along neuronal axons (conductive fibers that comprise the information pathways of the brain and the peripheral nerves of the body). Upon reaching the target cell, these electrical signals generate small synaptic potentials. Such local changes in the voltage across the membrane of a target cell add or subtract voltage to the intrinsic oscillation of the target cell receiving the signal. Intrinsic oscillatory properties and modifying synaptic potentials are the coinage that a neuron uses to arrive at the generation of its own action potential message, which it will send on to other neurons or to muscle fibers. And so, in the case of muscle, all possible behaviors in us arise from activation of the motor neurons that activate the muscles that ultimately orchestrate our movements. These motor neurons in turn receive messages from other neurons located "up stream" from them (figure 1.2).

The peaks and valleys of the electrical oscillations of neurons can dictate the waxing and waning of a cell's responsiveness to incoming synaptic signals. It may determine at any moment in time whether the cell chooses to "hear" and respond to an incoming electrical signal or ignore it altogether. As will be discussed in more depth in chapter 4, this oscillatory switching of electrical activity is not only very important in neuron-to-neuron communication and whole network function, it is the electrical glue that allows the brain to organize itself functionally and architecturally during development. Indeed, simultaneity of neuronal activity is the most pervasive mode of operation of the brain, and neuronal oscillation provides the means for this simultaneity to occur in a predictable, if not continuous, manner.

Coherence Rhythmicity and Resonance   Neurons that display rhythmic oscillatory behavior may entrain to each other via action potentials. The resulting, far-reaching consequence of this is neuronal groups that oscillate in phase—that is, coherently, which supports simultaneity of activity.

Consider the issue of coherence from the perspective of communication, for coherence is what communication rides on. Imagine a soft summer night in a rural setting. Amidst the rich quietude, you hear first one cicada, then another. Soon, there are many chirping. More importantly, they may chirp in rhythmic unison (note that to chirp in unison they must all have a similar internal clock that tells them when to chirp next—such a mechanism is known as an intrinsic oscillator). The first cicada may be calling out to see if there are any kin about. But this unison of many cicadas chirping rhythmically becomes a bonding, literally a conglomerated functional state. In the subtle fluctuations of this rhythmicity comes the transfer of information, at the whole community level, to a vast number of remotely located individuals. Similar events occur in

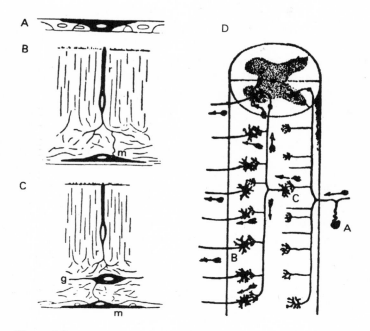

Figure 1.2

Evolution of nervous systems. An interneuron, in the strict sense, is any nerve cell that does not communicate directly with the outside world either as a sensing device (a sensory neuron) or by means of a motor terminal on a muscle (a motor neuron). Interneurons, therefore, receive and send information to other nerve cells exclusively. Their evolution and development represent the basis for the elaboration of the central nervous system. The diagrams above represent stages of development present in early invertebrates. In (*A*), a motile cell (in black) from a primitive organism (a sponge), responds to direct stimulation with a wave of contraction. In (*B*), in more evolved primitive organisms (e.g., the sea anemone), the sensory and contractile functions of the cell in A have been segregated into two elements; "r" is the receptor or sensory cell and "m" is the muscle or contractile element. The sensory cell responds to stimuli and serves as a motor neuron in the sense that it triggers muscle-cell contraction. However, this sensory cell has become specialized so that it is incapable of generating movement (contraction) on its own. Its function at this stage is the reception and transmission of information. In (*C*), a second neuron has been interposed between the sensory element and the muscle (also from a sea anemone). This cell, a motor neuron, serves to activate muscle fibers (m) but responds only to the activation of the sensory cell (r) (Parker 1919). In (*D*), as the evolution of the central nervous system progresses (this example is the vertebrate spinal cord), cells become interposed between the sensory neurons (A) and motor neurons (B). These are the interneurons, which serve to distribute the sensory information (arrow in A) by their many branches (arrows in C) to the motor neurons or to other neurons in the central nervous system. (Adapted from Ramón y Cajal, 1911.)

some types of fireflies, which synchronize their light flash activity and may illuminate trees in a blinking fashion like Christmas tree lights.

This effect of oscillating in phase so that scattered elements may work together as one in an amplified fashion is known as resonance—and neurons do it, too. In fact, a local group of neurons resonating in phase with each other may then resonate with another group of neurons that are quite far from the first group (Llinás 1988; Hutcheon and Yarom 2000). Electrical resonance, a property supported by direct electrical connectivity among cells (as occurs in the heart, allowing it to function as a pump by the simultaneous contraction of all of its component muscle fibers) is perhaps the oldest form of communication among neurons. The delicately detailed nuances of chemical synaptic transmission come later in evolution to enhance and embellish neuronal communication.

Not all neurons resonate at all times. It is the crucial property of neurons to be able to switch in and out of oscillatory modes of electrical activity that allows resonance to occur transiently among differing groups of neurons at different times. If they were not able to do this, they would not be able to represent the ever-changing reality that surrounds us. When differing groups of neurons capable of displaying oscillatory behavior "perceive" or encode different aspects of the same incoming signal, they may join their efforts by resonating in phase with each other. This is known as neuronal oscillatory coherence. Simultaneity of neuronal activity, brought into existence not by chance but by intrinsic oscillatory electrical activity, resonance, and coherence are, as we shall see, at the root of cognition. Indeed, such intrinsic activity forms the very foundation of the notion that there is such a thing called our "selves."

Returning to the original question of intrinsic properties, one may propose the following: that intrinsic electro-responsiveness of the brain's elements, the neurons and the networks they weave together, generate internal representations (connections) that engender functional states. These states are specified in detail, but not in context, by incoming sensory activity. That is, brain function is proposed to have two distinct components. One is the private or "closed" system that we have discussed and that is responsible for qualities such as subjectivity and semantics; the other is an "open" component responsible for sensory-motor transformations dealing with the relations between the private component and the external world (Llinás 1974, 1987). Because the brain operates for the most part as a closed system, it must be regarded as a reality emulator rather than a simple translator.

Acknowledging this, we might go on to say that the intrinsic electrical activity of the brain's elements (its neurons and their complex connectivity) must form an entity, or a functional construct. Furthermore, this entity must efficiently handle the transformation of sensory input arising from the external world into its motor output counterpart. How can we study such a complicated functional construct as this? First we must model it, make some assumptions concerning how the brain may be implementing such transformational properties, and for this we must be very clear about what the brain actually does. If we decide, as a working hypothesis, that this functional brain construct must bestow reality emulating properties, we may then consider what types of models could support such a function.

Let us begin with a simple sensory-motor transformation. The motor aspect is implemented by muscle force (contractile) exercised on bones linked to each other by hinges (joints). In order to study our assumed transformational properties, we may describe the contractile aspect as performing a given movement in space (or in mathematical terms, a vector), and so the set of all muscle contractions contributing to this movement (or any type of behavior) will be enacted in a "vectorial coordinate space." With this approach, the electrical activity patterns that each neuron generates in the formation of a motor pattern, or any other internal pattern in the brain, must be represented in an abstract geometric space. This is the vectorial coordinate space where sensory input and its transformation into a motor output take place (Pellionisz and Llinás 1982). If this sounds a bit like double-talk to you, please read the contents of box 1.1.

How Did the Mind Arise from Evolution?

Let us go back to the very first point made at the beginning of this chapter, that the mind did not just suddenly appear at some point fully formed. With some forethought and a little educated digging, we can find in biological evolution a quite convincing trail of clues as to the brain's

Box 1.1
Abstract Representation of Reality

Let us imagine a cube of electrically conductive material, a gelatin-like substance, held in a spherical glass aquarium. Let's imagine that the surface of the container has small electrical contacts that can allow electricity to pass between one contact and any other through the gelatin. Finally, let's say that the gelatin condenses into thin conductive filaments if current passes between the electrical contacts often, but returns to amorphous gel if no current flows for a while.

If we now pass current among some contacts connected to one or more sensory systems that transform a complex external state (let's say playing soccer) and other contacts related to a motor system, a condensed set of wirelike paths will grow that allows the sensory inputs to activate a motor output. (Keep in mind that these wires do not interact with each other—they are insulated, just as for the most part are the fiber pathways of the brain, and therefore there are no short circuits. These wires can, however, branch to generate a complex connectivity matrix). As we proceed to generate more complex sensory inputs they will in turn generate more complex motor outputs. In short, a jungle of "wires" grows inside the fishbowl, or melts, if stimuli are not repeated for a time. This veritable mess of wires would be the embedding that relates certain sensory inputs (in principle any thing that can be transduced by the senses, what we may call universals) to given motor outputs. As an example, this contraption could be used hypothetically to control a soccer-playing robot (backpropagation algorithms have this general form).

Looking at the fishbowl we can understand that there, somewhere in the complex geometry of wires, are the rules for playing soccer, but in a very different geometry from the playing of soccer itself. One cannot understand by direct inspection that the particular wiring represents such a thing. "Soccer" is being represented in a different geometry from that of soccer in external reality, and in an abstract geometry at that—no legs or referees or soccer balls, only wires. So the system is isomorphic (can enact soccer playing) although not homomorphic with soccer playing (does not look like soccer playing). This is analogous to the tape inside a videocassette, which despite close inspection offers no clues as to the details of the movie embedded in its magnetic code. Here we have a representation of the external world in which intrinsic coordinate systems operate to transform an input (a sensory event) into the appropriate output (a motor response) using the dynamic elements of the sensory organs and motor "plant," the set of all muscles and joints, or their equivalent. This sensory-motor transformation is the core of brain function, that is, what the brain does for a living.

origin. If one agrees that the mind and brain are one, then the evolution of this unique mindness function must certainly have coincided with the evolution of the nervous system itself. It should also be obvious that the forces driving the evolution of the nervous system shaped and determined the emergence of mind as well. The questions to ask here are clear. How and why did the nervous system evolve? What critical choices did nature have to make along the way?

It Began at a Critical Time

The first issue is whether a nervous system is actually necessary for all organized life beyond that of a single cell. The answer is no. Living organisms that do not move actively, including sessile organisms such as plants, have evolved quite successfully without a nervous system. And so we have landed our first clue: a nervous system is only necessary for multicellular creatures (not cell colonies) that can orchestrate and express active movement—a biological property known as "motricity." It is interesting to note that plants, which have well-organized circulatory systems but no hearts, appeared slightly later in evolution than did most primitive animals; it is as if sessile organisms had, in effect, chosen not to have a nervous system. Although this seems a rather strange statement to make, the facts are quite irrefutable—the Venus Flytrap, Mimosa, and other locally moving plants not withstanding.

Where does the story begin? What type of creature can we look to for support of this important connection between the early glimmerings of a nervous system and the actively moving, versus sessile, organism? A good place to begin is with the primitive *Ascidiacea*, tunicates or "sea squirts," which represent a fascinating juncture in our own early chordate (true backbone) ancestry (figure 1.3).

The adult form of this creature is sessile, rooted by its pedicle to a stable object in the sea (figure 1.4, left) (Romer 1969; Millar 1971; Cloney 1982). The sea squirt carries out two basic functions in its life: it feeds by filtering seawater, and it reproduces by budding. The larval form is briefly free-swimming (usually a day or less) and is equipped with a brainlike ganglion containing approximately 300 cells (Romer 1969; Millar 1971; Cloney 1992). This primitive nervous system receives sensory information about the surrounding environment through a statocyst

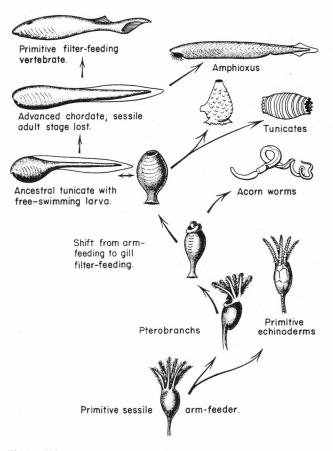

Primitive filter-feeding vertebrate.

Advanced chordate; sessile adult stage lost.

Ancestral tunicate with free-swimming larva.

Amphioxus

Tunicates

Acorn worms

Shift from arm-feeding to gill filter-feeding.

Pterobranchs

Primitive echinoderms

Primitive sessile arm-feeder.

Figure 1.3
A simplified diagram of chordate evolution. The tunicates, or sea squirts (*Ascidiaceae;* see figure 1.4) represents a stage in which the gill apparatus has become highly evolved in the sessile adult, while the larval stage in some species is free-swimming, exhibiting the advanced features of a notochord and nerve cord associated with the motile behavior. See text for more details. (Adapted from Romer, 1969, p. 30.)

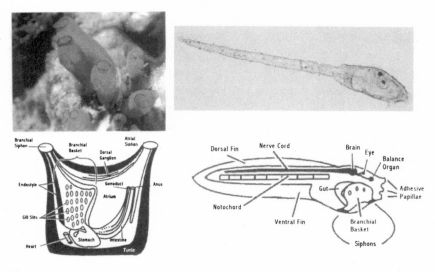

Figure 1.4
Sea squirts (*Ascidiaceae*) or tunicates, which have a sessile, filter-feeding adult stage attached to the substratum (*left*), and in many cases a brief free-swimming larval stage (*right*). (*Bottom left*) Diagram of a generalized adult solitary sea squirt. The black outer portion is its protective "tunic." (*Bottom right*) Diagram of a typical free-swimming sea squirt larva or tadpole. A gut, gills and branchial structure are present, but are neither functional nor open. See text for details. (From website www.animalnetwork.com/fish/aqfm/1997/)

(organ of balance), a rudimentary, light-sensitive patch of skin, and a notochord (primitive spinal cord) (figure 1.4, right). These features allow this tadpole-like creature to handle the vicissitudes of the ever-changing world within which it swims. Upon finding a suitable substrate (Svane and Young 1989; Young 1989; Stoner 1994), the larva proceeds to bury its head into the selected location and becomes sessile once again (Cloney 1982; Svane and Young 1989; Young 1989). Once reattached to a stationary object the larva absorbs—literally digests—most of its own brain, including its notochord. It also digests its tail and tail musculature, thereupon regressing to the rather primitive adult stage: sessile and lacking a true nervous system other than that required for activation of the simple filtering activity (Romer 1969; Millar 1971; Cloney 1982). The lesson here is quite clear: the evolutionary development of a nervous system is an exclusive property of actively moving creatures.

We have now derived a basic concept—namely, that brains are an evolutionary prerequisite for guided movement in primitive animals—and the reason for this becomes obvious. Clearly, active movement is dangerous in the absence of an internal plan subject to sensory modulation. Try walking any distance, even in a well-protected, uncluttered hallway, with your eyes closed. How far can you go before opening your eyes becomes irresistible? The nervous system has evolved to provide a plan, one composed of goal-oriented, mostly short-lived predictions verified by moment-to-moment sensory input. This allows a creature to move actively in a direction according to an internal reckoning—a transient sensorimotor image—of what may be outside. The next question in our pursuit of the evolution of mind should now be clear. How did the nervous system evolve to be able to perform the sophisticated task of prediction?

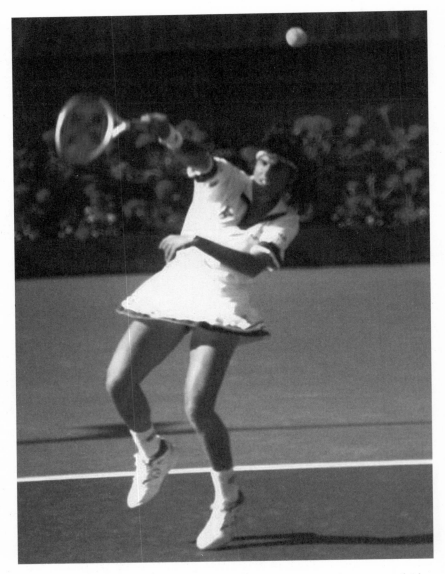

Tennis pro Gabriella Sabatini returns a shot. Photo reprinted courtesy of Alan Cook, alcook@sprintmail.com, http://alancook.50mpegs.com.

2

Prediction Is the Ultimate Function of the Brain

Why Must the Brain Predict?

In chapter 1, we argued that a nervous system is only necessary for living creatures that move actively. If so, how has a nervous system contributed to their evolutionary success? Clearly, such creatures must move intelligently in order to survive, to procure food and shelter, and to avoid becoming food for someone else. I use the word "intelligently" to imply that a creature must employ a rudimentary strategy, or at the very least rely upon a set of tactical rules regarding the basic properties of the external world through which it moves. Otherwise, movement would be purposeless and necessarily dangerous. The creature must anticipate the outcome of a given movement on the basis of incoming sensory stimuli. A change in its immediate environment must evoke a movement (or lack of it) in response to ensure survival. The capacity to predict the outcome of future events—critical to successful movement—is, most likely, the ultimate and most common of all global brain functions.

Before proceeding, it is important to have a clear sense of what is meant by "prediction." Prediction is a forecast of what is likely to occur. For example, we predict common outcomes—such as walking barefooted on the hot pavement will hurt, or that not turning the car when approaching a dead-end will result in something probably harmful to you and the car. When one runs to hit a tennis ball, one must predict where in time and space the ball and the face of one's racket can successfully meet.

Consider two mountain rams squaring to fight. As they eye one another, they slowly rise onto their hind legs and look for the tiniest of clues that will provide a hint of when the other is about to shift its weight forward and charge. Because even a half-step lead in momentum can change the outcome of the contest, a ram (or any creature for that matter) must be able to anticipate the attack in order to counter strike, that is, it must be able to predict that a blow is coming before it arrives.

The ability to predict is critical in the animal kingdom—a creature's life often depends upon it. Still, the mechanism of prediction is far more ubiquitous in the brain's control of body function than the examples so far described. Consider the simple act of reaching for a carton of milk in the refrigerator. Without giving much focused thought to our action, we must predict the carton's weight, its slipperiness, its degree of fullness, and, finally, the compensatory balance we must apply for a successfully smooth trajectory of the carton to our glass. Once movement is initiated, we adjust our movement and the compensatory balance as we receive direct sensory information coming in. However, before even reaching, we have made a ballpark, premotor prediction of what will be involved.

The brain's ability to predict is not only generated from our awareness of its operation; prediction is a far older evolutionary function than that. Consider this: have you ever found yourself blinking just before a bug lands in your eye? You did not see the bug, at least not on a conscious level, yet you anticipated the event and blinked appropriately to ward off its entry into your eye. Prediction is at the heart of this basic protective mechanism. Prediction, almost continually operative at conscious and reflex levels, is pervasive throughout most, if not all, levels of brain function.

In the beginning of this book, I mentioned that the mindness state, which may or may not necessarily represent external reality, has evolved as a goal-oriented device to guide the interactions between a living organism and its environment. Success in a goal-oriented, moving system is enhanced by an innate mechanism for prediction. Furthermore, we can assume that prediction must be grounded, that there can be only one predictive organ. It would make little sense if the head predicted one thing and the tail another. Predictive functions must be centralized.

Prediction and the Origin of "Self"

Although prediction is localized in the brain, it does not occur at only one site in the brain. These predictive functions must be brought together into a single understanding or construct; otherwise, the end result would be no different than if prediction were grounded in any number of different organs. What pulls these functions together? What is the repository of predictive function? I believe the answer lies in what we call the self: *self is the centralization of prediction.* The self is not born out of the realm of consciousness, only the noticing of it is (i.e., self-awareness). According to this view, the self can exist without awareness of its own existence. Even in we as self-aware individuals, self-awareness is not continuously present. In the middle of a difficult challenge, such as swimming away from a shark, you will try to get to shore and be quite aware of what is happening, but you will probably not be thinking to yourself, "Here I am swimming away from a shark." You will think about it only when you get to shore and safety.

The concept of self-awareness will be discussed in later chapters, but I wanted to point to the issue of self now. Understanding that the brain performs prediction on the basis of an assumed self "entity" will lead us to how the brain generates the mindness state.

Why this predictive ability arose is clear: it is critical to survival, guiding it at the level of both the single animal (moment-to-moment) and the species (in fact, of all actively moving species throughout evolution). How did the ability to predict arise from evolution? The answer can be found with a little thoughtful digging. First, however, we must understand how the nervous system actually performs prediction; once we know that, we will find the answer to how nature evolved this amazing function.

As we will see later in this chapter, for the nervous system to predict, it must perform a rapid comparison of the sensory-referred properties of the external world with a separate internal sensorimotor representation of those properties. For the prediction to be useful, the nervous system must then transform or utilize this premotor solution into finely timed and executed movement. Once a pattern of neural activity acquires internal significance (sensory content gains internal context), the brain generates a strategy of what to do next—another pattern of neural activity. This strategy can be considered an internal representation of what is to come. Such premotor patterns of neural activity must then be transformed into the neuronal activity that sets into motion the appropriate bodily movement: These transformations require an internal representation of what is to come, in order for them to become actualized in the external world context (figure 2.1).

Prediction Saves Time and Effort   Prediction is crucial to brain function not only for the successful execution of goal-oriented, active movement, but also as a basic functional operation in order to conserve time and energy. This may sound a bit strange, since the nervous system—particularly the human nervous system—being the most sophisticated and capable "processor" yet known, might be expected to be above such trivial considerations. Nevertheless, when the brain deals with the vicissitudes of the external world (and the internal as well) its activity does not parallel reality in its continuity; it just feels that way to us. In real life the brain operates in a discontinuous manner from a processing perspective. It is not possible to take in all of the information available to our senses from the external world and then arrive at the correct decision quickly in a continuous fashion. Neurons are fast, but they are not that fast. Note, I am still only speaking of the premotor phase of processing. Remember that a successful interaction with the external world also necessitates the subsequent timely execution of the brain's given decision through movement.

It seems that the brain must compartmentalize incoming information and implement its attention on a need to know basis in order to fuel its momentary decision-making ability without overloading. The brain must leave itself enough time to implement a movement decision so that it remains in step with what is happening in the external world at a given moment. It must also be able to skip to the next moment's need for processing without being encumbered by the previous moment's processing. In other words, the brain cannot be stuck doing one thing when it needs to move on to the next task. This mode of operation derives from what is known as a look ahead function, which is an inherent property of

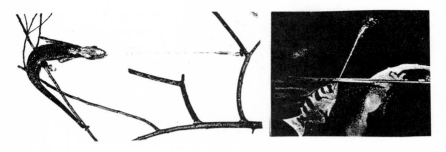

Figure 2.1
Two examples of the ability of animals to plan motor execution by predicting events to come. (*Left*) A chameleon midway in the process of extending and withdrawing its sticky-tipped tongue to capture an insect. (*Right*) The archer fish of the East Indies, so named because it rapidly and accurately shoots drops of water to stun and capture insects or spiders near the water's surface. (Photographs courtesy of the New York Zoological Society. Adapted from Romer, 1969, pp. 68 and 167.)

neuronal circuits. Indeed, prediction begins at the single neuron level. We can address this issue with an example: the control of movement.

Prediction and the Control of Movement

Because the ability to predict evolved in tandem with increasingly complex movement strategies, we must look at movement control in order to understand prediction. Let us return to the refrigerator for a carton of milk. The appropriate pattern of contraction must be specified for an extension/grasping sequence to be executed properly (add to this the correct use of postural muscles for support of the body while bending over during the reach). Now consider what the brain must do to pull off this simple movement sequence. Each muscle provides a direction of pull (a vector). Each muscle vector is composed of individual muscle fibers that are operated in pre-established groups based on their common innervation by the same motor neuron. This is called a motor unit (a single motor neuron innervates tens to hundreds of muscle fibers). A given muscle may be composed of hundreds of such individual motor units. The number of muscles multiplied by the number of motor units may then be viewed as the total number of degrees of freedom for any given movement. A movement such as reaching into the refrigerator is considered a simple one (as compared to, say, a good tennis return). However, from a functional perspective, even a simple movement often engages most of the body's muscles, resulting in an astronomical number of possible simultaneous and/or sequential muscle contractions and degrees of freedom. With the milk carton example, your arm may be brought toward the carton from any number of initial positions and postures (maybe your back hurts today and so you bend into your reach from a stilted, atypical stance).

All of this potential complexity exists before the load is actually placed on your arm and body; you have yet to pick up the carton and can only guess its weight during your initial reaching motion.

So this simple movement is not simple when we break it down and try to understand how the brain handles it all. However, the dimensionality of the problem of motor control does not derive solely from the number of muscles involved, the differing degrees of pull force and angle, and so forth. The real dimensionality of the problem stems from the complicated interaction between the possible directions of muscle pull and their sequence of activation in time.

Much of motor control occurs in real time, "on-line," as it were. Our movements seldom take place under stimulus-free conditions. Consider the following scenarios: running down a steep, winding forest path; steering your car while holding a cup of coffee; jumping up and stretching to return a serve in tennis. The combination of muscles one contracts at any given moment is often determined as a movement sequence and executed in response to teleceptive stimuli (stimuli at a distance taken in mainly through the senses of hearing and vision), kinesthetic feedback (the feeling of one's body moving), or thought.

It is generally assumed that the optimal controller is one that produces the smoothest possible movement. This idea implies the continuous monitoring (that is to say, a sampling rate of every millisecond or faster) of feed-forward and feedback influences on the selected activation sequences in order to minimize the accelerative transients that produce jerkiness in movement. Although this sounds right, we need to evaluate whether it is computationally plausible for the brain to control movement in such a continuous, on-line manner.

From the heuristic formula described above, and, given that there are 50 or so key muscles in the hand, arm, and shoulder that one uses to reach for the milk carton, over 10^{15} combinations of muscle contractions are possible—a staggering number to say the least. If during every millisecond of this reaching/grasping sequence the single best of the 10^{15} combinations is chosen after an evaluation of all of the possibilities, then 10^{18} decisions would have to be made every second. This would mean that the brain, if it were a computer, would need a 1-exahertz (1 million gigahertz) processor to choose the correct muscle combinations to execute appropriately this relatively simple reaching/grasping sequence. In reality, even the above scenario is an over simplification (Welsh et al. 1995). The dimensionality of the problem of motor control is increased many orders of magnitude when one also considers that there is a bare minimum of 100 motor units for every muscle, and that each muscle pull may, and most likely will, involve differing sets of motor neurons.

The brain does not seem to have evolved to deal with the control of movement in this fashion—especially when one considers that there are on the order of 10^{11} neurons in the entire brain. Of these, only a fraction are in the cerebellum, the area of brain where most of the movement control processing would take place for the movement sequence we have been discussing (Llinás and Simpson 1981).

An alternative solution for the continuous control of movement might be a scheme where each muscle in the body is somehow controlled independently through time. Metaphorically, the motor system could be considered a bank of discrete representations (or parallel processors, with one for each muscle). This set-up would significantly ease the functional burden for the control of any single muscle, and render trivial the problem of how to control a highly artificial and rare movement involving only one or two muscles. This scenario presents significant difficulties for the control of complicated muscle synergies, however. A muscle synergy is a set of muscles working in tandem to bring about a given movement. This synergy operates on the stretch reflex, that is, the relation between flexors and extensors (figure 2.2). For instance, our reaching for the milk carton sequence is a muscle synergy, as are the associated muscles involved in the ensuing grasping movement of our hand and the reflex properties of the spinal cord circuits. As the number of muscles involved in a movement sequence increases, there would be a greater reliance on an absolutely precise and infallible synchronizing element to ensure that the muscle activations occur cohesively in time.

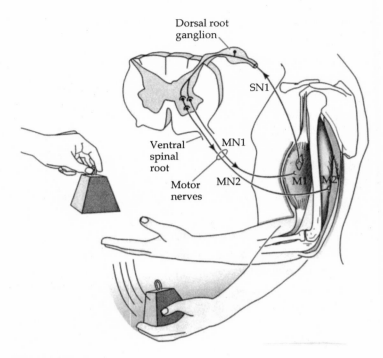

Figure 2.2
Example of the stretch reflex circuit. When a load is placed in the hand, the stretch receptor in the biceps flexor muscle sends a signal to the spinal cord that triggers the stimulation of the biceps muscle and the inhibition of its opposing extensor, the triceps muscle. The result is maintenance or recovery of arm position with the added weight. The entire reflex circuit is contained within the spinal cord and periphery. (From Rosenzweig et al. 1999, figure 11.10.)

This solution seems more fitting for a digital computer than a nervous system. However, unlike the elements of a digital system, neurons are analog: they have nonlinear response properties, and do not fire their action potentials with sufficient temporal precision to control continuously in time such parallel processing machinery.

At this point it should be clear that the continuous control of movement through time demands an extremely high computational overhead. This is true whether the movement is controlled by regulating the activity of every muscle discretely in parallel, or by choosing and implementing combinations of muscles. We do, of course, make complicated movements, and quite often. To delve further into this issue, we must ask the following:

1. How might the dimensionality problem of motor control, this incredible functional overhead for the brain, be reduced without significantly degrading the quality of movement sequences?
2. Which well-established aspects of brain function can provide clues for how to solve this problem?

The Discontinuous Nature of Movement

A relatively straightforward approach to reducing the dimensionality of motor control for the brain is to decrease the temporal resolution of the controlling system, that is, remove it from the burden of being continuously on-line and processing. This can be accomplished by breaking up the time line of the motor task into a series of smaller units over which the controller must operate. Control would be discontinuous in time and thus the operations of such a system would occur at discrete intervals of a "dt" (literally, intervals of a discrete passage of time). We must here consider an important consequence, that movements controlled by this type of pulsatile system would not be executed continuously, demonstrating obligatorily smooth kinematics, but rather would be executed in a discontinuous fashion as a linked series of muscle twitches. Motor physiologists have known this fact for over a century: movements are not executed continuously, but are discontinuous in nature. E. A. Schafer surmised this as early as 1886:

The curve of a voluntary muscular contraction . . . invariably shows, both at the commencement of the contraction and during its continuance, a series of undulations that succeed one another with almost exact regularity, and can, as it would seem, only be interpreted to indicate the rhythm of the muscular response to the voluntary stimuli which provoke the contraction. . . . The undulations . . . are plainly visible and are sufficiently regular in size and succession to leave no doubt in the mind of any person who has seen a graphic record of muscular tetanic contraction produced by exciting the nerve about 10 times in the second, that the curve . . . is that of a similar contraction. (9)

A tetanic contraction, or tetanus, is the maximum force that a muscle can generate when activated at high frequency. Schafer realized that a clearly defined rhythmicity in the range of 8–12 Hz exists in volitional muscular contraction. Following Schafer's initial report, the phenomenon of an 8–12 Hz periodicity to voluntary movement, termed "physiological tremor," became a topic of intense research. In 1894, Harris measured the frequency of the "voluntary tetanus" (literally, the voluntary driving of a muscle or muscle synergy to its maximum rhythmic speed, as in flexing and extending one's finger as quickly as possible, or the maximum rate at which one can voluntarily shake a foot, etc.) in a variety of muscles, including those of the arm, hand, fingers, and tongue. Discontinuities of 8–12 Hz were observed in all of the muscles he studied.

Harris went on to state that "the average rate of single voluntary muscle twitches is 10 or 11 per second—a figure sufficiently near to that of the rate of the voluntary tetanus as to be reckoned identical with it." In essence, what is seen at the single muscle level is reflected in the overt movement. In 1910, Sherrington noted that the scherzo of Schubert's *Piano Quartet No. 8* requires repetitive hand movements at approximately 8 Hz, which approaches the upper limit for finger movements by professional pianists. He also observed that the syllable "la" cannot be repeated more than 11 times per second and went on to state that "the limit set to the frequency of repetition of the same one movement seems to be 11 per second."

Some years later, Travis (1929) demonstrated that voluntary movement initiated from a holding position was almost always initiated in phase with physiological tremor. He reported that "a voluntary movement is, in most instances, a continuation of tremor . . . [it] does not interrupt the tremor rhythm . . . and fits into the kinetic melody" determined by the brain. Travis went on to suggest that the maximum rate of a repeated voluntary movement could not exceed the rate of physiological tremor. More recently, the study of physiological tremor has brought to light what may be a very close relationship between the close to 10-Hz rhythmic discontinuity and the actual onset of movement itself. The work of Travis was advanced in 1956, when Marshall and Walsh demonstrated that the reflection of external movements in humans does indeed start at the phase of the physiological tremor corresponding to the direction of the intended movement.

These researchers also noted that the physiological discontinuities in voluntary movements were independent of both the velocity of the movement and the load imposed on the limb. In essence, although the maximum rate for a voluntary repetitive movement cannot exceed the rate of physiological tremor in the muscle, the tremor rhythm exists, unchanged in its periodicity, regardless of the speed of the overt movement or whether or not there is any force acting on the muscle. In the last 15 years or so, it has become clear that the 8–12 Hz rhythmicity of physiological tremor is observed not only during voluntary movement, but also, and perhaps to a greater extent, during maintained posture and in supported limbs at rest (Marsden et al. 1984).

Most recently, Wessberg, Vallbo, and colleagues (1995; Vallbo and Wessberg 1993; Wicklund Fernstrom et al. 1999) found prominent 8–10 Hz discontinuities in slow and "smooth" finger movements (figure 2.3). As the latencies of the stretch reflex contributing to these movements were incompatible with the timing of the observed discontinuities of the movements, they suggested (Wessberg and Vallbo 1995) that such discontinuities were most likely generated from brain levels above the spinal cord. The stretch reflex is a simple, negative feedback mechanism involving a muscle fiber and its associated segmental spinal cord circuitry; when a muscle is passively stretched this compensatory reflex causes a subsequent contraction. From the latency of this reflex (from stretch to contraction) that these authors calculated, they were able to conclude that the reflex could not explain the timing of the tremor components seen in the above study. Hence, Wessberg and Vallbo (1995) suggested that the drive causing these periodic components must derive from brain structures higher than the spinal cord.

N. A. Bernstein asked more than 30 years ago (1967), "Is there no reason to suppose that this [tremor] frequency marks the appearance of rhythmic oscillations in the excitability of all, or of the main elements of the . . . motor apparatus, in which a mutual synchronization through rhythm is doubtless necessary?"

We see that the underlying nature of movement is not as smooth and continuous as our voluntary movements appear; rather, the execution of movement is a discontinuous series of muscle twitches, the periodicity of

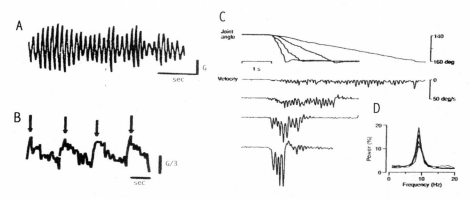

Figure 2.3
Examples of tremor. (*A, B*) Tracing of wrist flexion and extension in a normal adult showing movement rhythmicity at 10 Hz (Schäfer 1886). (*C*) Sample records to demonstrate a subject's performance in voluntary ramps of varying velocities. Upper records in (*A*) show angular displacement and lower records the corresponding angular velocities. The track speeds were 4, 10, 25, and 62 degrees/second. (*D*) Power spectra from 160 records of the same subject when tracking the same four track speeds. Single peak is at 8–10 Hz. (From Vallbo and Wessberg, 1993, figure 4, p. 680).

which is highly regular. Furthermore, this physiological tremor is apparent even at rest (when we are not actively making movements). Indeed, the tremor is highly associated with movement onset and movement direction. For instance, upward movements are initiated during the ascending phase of physiological tremor (Goodman and Kelso 1983).

What do these rhythmic discontinuities represent? What might be their functional significance? To understand this, we may invoke the principle of parsimony (Occam's Razor). So what is the simplest answer that will fit the data?

Perhaps the most parsimonious explanation is one that takes into account the unbelievably high functional overhead the brain must handle in the control of movement. From the example above, it appears that these rhythmic discontinuities are not an inherent property of muscle tissue itself, but rather that this physiological tremor might be a reflection, at the musculoskeletal level, of a descending command from the forebrain that is pulsatile in nature. If the control system operates discontinuously (to avoid high computational overhead), a pulsatile nature is ideal. Although this is a step in the right direction for lowering our functional overhead, without gaining something in return, the risk of running motor control discontinuously could easily lead to choppy movements, with the uncertainty of whether muscle groups will synchronize appropriately in time through the execution of a given movement. What else might be gained by pulsatile control through time, apart from easing up on the brain's workload?

Motor Binding in Time and the Centralization of Prediction

A pulsatile input into motor neurons from a control system, as opposed to a command system, may prepare a population of independent motor neurons for a descending command by uniformly biasing these motor neurons into their linear range of responsivity (Greene 1972). To clarify, a pulsatile control input would serve to "linearize" a population of nonlinear and independent neuronal elements in order to ensure a uniform population response to a command signal. The motor neurons that need to be recruited for a given movement are often separated by many spinal levels; this pulsatile mechanism may serve as a cueing function to synchronize such motor neuronal activities.

A pulsatile control system might also allow for brief periods of movement acceleration in order to provide an inertial break mechanism to overcome frictional forces and the viscosity of muscles (Goodman and Kelso 1983). For example, when we rock a snowbound car, this type of movement helps to extract it.

Finally, a periodic control system may allow for input and output to be bound in time. In other words, this type of control system might enhance the ability of sensory inputs and descending motor commands to be integrated within the functioning motor apparatus as a whole.

What then is the difference between a controller system and a command system? A controller system sends only the necessary (need to know) orders for each one of the elements of the system to execute a global command (it micromanages). A command system, on the other hand, gives the same global instructions at the same time to all involved ("Get it done—I don't care how"). It is clear that these systems must work together: everybody standing around with no idea of what to do is like a union without work; a well-defined project with none of the key workers on hand is a project undone. If you want to understand the workings of the brain, the division of labor metaphor is often the most illuminating. The only difference is the time frame. The brain operates in the millisecond domain, requiring an agility that provides self-reorganizing of focus at the drop of a hat.

For right now, I want to focus on the control system. Later, we shall deal with the command system, although we have already indicated that the command system is the self (i.e., the centralization of prediction).

We have begun to describe conceptually the way the brain lessens the work it must do in motor control. We now understand that operating continuously online, which we might have thought was the only way the brain could bring about smoothly executed movement, is simply not possible physiologically. Instead, the brain has relegated the rallying of the motor troops to the control of a pulsatile, discontinuous-in-time signal, which is reflected in the musculoskeletal system as physiological tremor. Other than just saving the brain from being computationally overwhelmed, a pulsatile control input also serves to bring the neurons, muscles, or limbs closer to a threshold for some action, be it firing, integration, or movement. The possible risks of operating discontinuously in time are beautifully minimized by the synchronizing effect this pulsatile signal has on the independent elements, at all levels, of the motor apparatus. Let us remember the words of Bernstein: "a mutual synchronization through rhythm is doubtless necessary" for the motor apparatus as a whole.

Before pressing on with this conceptual investigation of how the functional overhead of motor control may be lessened, I would like to touch on something else. Today we know that a physiological tremor is a reflection, at the musculoskeletal level, of a descending control signal (the nature and source of which we shall discuss shortly). Yet, during early stages of development, the tremor is not just a reflection. In fact, *the tremor is a property inherent to and exclusive of muscle tissue* (Harris and Whiting 1954). This is known as the myogenic moment of motricity, which occurs during development before motoneurons have even made contact with the muscles they will later drive. In the next chapter, we shall see how this tremor is "handed" from the muscles to the motoneurons that innervate them, and then to the upper motoneurons that drive them, and further and further "inward" to become the controller system and, ultimately the command system. I shall state again what I have said from the outset: *that which we call thinking is the evolutionary internalization of movement.*

Synergies Save Time

Let us return again to the issue of reducing the dimensionality of the problem of motor control for the brain. We understand now that this controller system operates discontinuously in time and eases the network burden brought about by being continuously on-line. Would it not also help in this regard to have the brain control muscles as discrete collectives instead of individually? A muscle collective is a group of muscles that are activated simultaneously—as in our grasping movement for the carton of milk. A muscle collective, or a time series of muscle collectives, that is successful in achieving some purpose is a muscle synergy. I referred to synergies earlier, but consider this: if the target units controlled by the brain are collectives or synergies rather than the individual muscles themselves, the brain's functional load underlying their control will be greatly reduced. The extent of this reduction will be proportional to the degree to which subsets of muscles are activated simultaneously in a given movement execution. Controlling muscle collectives rather than single muscles reduces the number of degrees of freedom and thereby simplifies the underlying computation needed for control.

The early studies of complex reflexes helped to explain that the brain may control movement through muscle collectives rather than through the control of individual muscles. One such example is the vestibulospinal reflex, the mechanism by which you automatically correct your body position when you begin to lose your equilibrium (if riding a bicycle, lean when turning!). Such reflexes engage collections of muscles that span multiple joints and are innervated by motoneurons from many different spinal levels (Brooks 1983). The stereotyped and time-locked performance of multiple, clearly independent muscles in these reflexes suggested to early researchers that the muscles were activated by a single command and controlled as a single, functional entity. The idea implied that a relatively invariant coupling of muscle activities underlies the performance of certain complex movements.

Actually, when we think of all the movements we make—or are capable of making—most are not composed of such stereotypic, hard-wired patterns of muscular activation. Furthermore, most complex voluntary (as opposed to reflex) movements can be executed successfully in a great number of ways—ways that may involve different combinations of muscles. For instance, maybe you will grab the carton of milk from its left side on one occasion and from the opposite side on another. This, however, does not invalidate the claim that muscle collectives need to save time and energy. Considering that muscle synergies and collectives may well underlie movement may help us reorient, heuristically, our views on the neuronal organization of motor control.

We see that muscles are often used in combinations, that fixed or hard-wired synergies are not the only rule, and that muscle combinations clearly change dynamically—as they must—during the execution of a complex movement. If muscle collectives, not individual muscles, are the units to be controlled, then what does this ask of the central process underlying the control of movement? It demands that as a complex movement proceeds, the control system must be able to reconfigure itself dynamically so that these collectives are cast temporarily, quickly dissolved, and rearranged as required. Because the central nervous system has many possible solutions for a given motor task, it follows that any given functional synergy organized by the brain must be a fleeting, dissipative construct. Furthermore, such constructs may not be easily recognized in behavior as an invariant pattern of muscle activation such as those we recognize in many overt, stereotypical reflexes.

If one postulates an "over complete" system of muscle collectives, this would ensure a degree of versatility and flexibility in choices that the control system could make. If we think of all the different ways we can reach for the milk carton, the idea of over-completeness is clear. If the motor control system may select from an over complete pool of similar functional synergies, any number of which get the job done reasonably well, then this would certainly lower the burden for the control system. It would ease the demand for precision, for having to make the right choice every time.

Doing the Two-Step

To continue with this train of thought, one may propose that the execution of rapid voluntary movements consists of two components with differing forms of operation. The first component is a feedforward, ballistic (no modulation *en route)* approximation of the movement's endpoint (get your hand close to the carton of milk) in which only advance sensory information can be used to shape the initial trajectory of a movement (open loop). In other words, we see the milk carton before we reach for it, and this sensory information is fed forward to the premotor control system to help it choose an appropriate reaching movement we should then make. The second component fine tunes the movement. This component operates "closed loop," meaning that it allows for sensory feedback to refine the movement as it is being executed, using tactile, kinesthetic, vestibular (balance), or visual cues (get a hold of the carton). Feedback fine tuning allows us to alter the trajectory of our reaching motion if we happen to hit, mistakenly, the door or the ketchup bottle with our hand, and similarly to make motion adjustments once we have grasped the carton based on its now known weight and slipperiness. For these reasons, feedforward control is sometimes referred to as predictive, while feedback control is sometimes referred to as reflective.

Greene (1982) suggests that the synergy underlying the feedforward component of a complex voluntary movement is selected from a variety of ballpark estimates that will approximate, but not precisely render, the desired endpoint. In this scheme, the magnitude of the feedback adjustment of the movement is inversely proportional to the precision with which the feedforward contribution can achieve the desired endpoint. Selecting a more optimal muscle synergy for the task will reduce the amount of follow-up effort required to correct any deviation produced by the feedforward component. Keep in mind, however, that if only one muscle synergy can approximate the desired movement endpoint, an erroneous selection would require a large correction with loss of time and of movement coordination. But as I said before, because there are many synergies to choose from that will approximate the desired movement, due to their over completeness, this reduces the necessity for an absolutely precise selection. As long as the selection is within the ballpark, the savings from operating in a feedforward mode will pay for the minimal follow-up effort based on feedback.

Lastly, the dimensionality of the problem of motor control can be reduced yet further if the motor system selects away from muscle collectives that are meaningless or maladaptive to prevent pollution of its pool of choices. Meaningless muscle synergies impose a great deal of extra work on the motor system, as feedback modulation to bring the movement to its desired endpoint would be at a premium. The selection of useful synergies requires an innate mechanism for biasing the motor system toward meaningful muscle collectives. In chapter 3, when we look into how the brain's ability to predict arose from evolution, the formation of meaningful muscle collectives will be as clear as why there is only one seat of prediction: survival is not random.

Summarizing So Far

Before looking more deeply into the control of movement and its intimate relationship with the predictive properties of the brain, let us look back and summarize to this point.

We have discussed two fundamental reasons why the brain must perform prediction. First, at the behavioral level any actively moving creature must have predictive abilities in order to interact with the external world in a meaningful way. Second, without intelligent and rapid interaction with the external world via active movement, life for such creatures would be necessarily more dangerous than it already is.

We understood that prediction at this level occurs by the formation—indeed, formulation—of a sensorimotor image, a contextualization of the external world. This internal, premotor image of what is to come is referenced to the properties of the external world as reported by sensory mechanisms such as hearing, vision, or touch. The solution to this comparison of internal and external worlds is then externalized: an appropriate action is taken, a movement is made. By this process a spectacular transference has occurred: an "upgrading" of the internal image of what is to come to its actualization into the external world.

We also came to understand that prediction must be centralized so that the premotor/sensorimotor images formed by the predictive properties are understood as a single construct. This is actually the issue of cognitive binding, and the neural mechanisms that formulate single, cognitively bound constructs are the same as those that generate, as a single construct, the subconscious sensorimotor image that says close your eye, a bug is coming.

The second reason that the brain must operate by prediction is to conserve energy for lessening the enormous burden of movement control. It has become clear that although movements seem smooth and continuous to us in their execution, they are not: they are generated and controlled discontinuously through time, in a pulsatile fashion, at discrete intervals of a dt look-ahead function. This highly periodic control signal is reflected in our muscles as the 8–12 Hz physiological tremor, which occurs both during movement and at rest. This pulsatile, premotor control signal saves time and computational overhead by not being continuously online. It also serves to synchronize all the elements of the motor apparatus so that these elements can all hear the command signal and thus operate as a single construct, the timely execution of a given movement.

We saw that the brain also saves time by using muscle collectives rather than individual muscles as the target units to control. Computational energy is further conserved by an over-complete pool of functional synergies to choose from for the initial stage of a rapid, voluntary movement, thus keeping costly feedback control to a minimum. The controller system has many functional muscle synergies that will reasonably approximate a movement endpoint, and this saves the system time by not forcing it to choose the precise functional synergy. Lastly, the motor system only allows for the formation of synergies that will get the job done as efficiently as possible, further lowering computational overhead.

A common thread emerges from all we have discussed so far. In order for the brain to predict, as when I move my tennis racket in space and time to successfully hit the ball, the brain must be capable of rapid and dramatic reorganization of focus. Moreover, when we think in such terms, it becomes clear that at any point in time the brain operates on a what-is-important-to-know-at-this-moment-only basis. There is no choice really; the brain has no time for anything else! In similar fashion the brain operates as a reality emulator, a generator of conscious experience. In order to deliver a reconstruction of the external world that is a seamless, dreamlike movie flowing continuously through time, it must forever be anticipating or looking ahead, operating and orienting its focus discontinuously in time, piecing it all together while jumping in discrete intervals of time. One can see that prediction drives this dissipative, fast reorganizing of focus. How the brain calls up, employs, and then dissolves muscle synergies on its need-to-know (or use) basis and how this reorganizing of focus occurs at the conscious level are one and the same: it would be a strange brain if it used different global strategies for motion and cognition. In the last sections of this chapter, I aim to de-mystify why this is so.

How Can a Neuronal Circuit Predict? A More Detailed View

Taking what we have learned thus far, it is time to turn up the magnification of our microscope and look a bit closer. We must investigate how our motor controller system does what it does: how it actually controls our movements discontinuously through time. From there we will be able to understand the nature of consciousness, and that its generation is discontinuous in time as well. First, however, we must understand how it is that a neural circuit actually predicts.

Two decades ago, Andras Pellionisz and I tried to determine how a neuronal circuit predicts (Pellionisz and Llinás 1979). We came to the conclusion that the brain predicts by taking advantage of the differences in electrical behavior among individual nerve cells. Because some neurons are highly sensitive to stimuli while others are less so, a dt look-ahead function might be implemented by neuronal circuits through a process analogous to a mathematical function known as the Taylor Series Expansion. This is the same dt we have been discussing all along. What this means in general terms is that those neurons that are very sensitive will tend to want to "jump the gun" or anticipate a given stimulus by responding to it before it is fully reformed. Rather than measuring how high a stimulus may be, these neurons respond to how fast a stimulus is changing. These "Nervous Nelly" neurons, by responding to the speed of

$\frac{dx}{dt}$ change of a stimulus, implement something similar to a mathematical differentiation: they respond faster than whatever it is that is changing in the outside world.

In the business world today, computer programs are beginning to predict fluctuations in the stock market by doing something very similar to what we proposed these highly responsive neurons do in the brain to generate prediction. As soon as a monitored stock begins to fall in value at a certain rate, the program implements a sell order; it does not wait for verification of what is happening. If the trend is reversed, it buys. If several computers are monitoring many different stocks, and they are carrying out this operation very quickly, they will make money. They respond not to the value but to the rate of change in value. Even though the programs allow gains of only very small increments, these small gains add up, and, what is more important, this way of operating will never let you crash.

Imagine that there are many computers in parallel, each simultaneously taking different measurements of an event in the external world. If some are extrapolating quickly, some doing so at intermediate velocities, and finally, some measuring the event in real time, what one ends up with is a reconstruction of the event ahead of its time of completion. This is the dt look-ahead function. Neuronal circuits do this. For example, one closes one's eye before the insect can land in it by extrapolating that at its estimated speed of approach, the insect will land in the open eye very shortly. The result: the eye is shut before the insect gets to it.

The same mechanism operates when you are playing tennis: you swing the racket to where you extrapolate the ball will be when the racket gets there, not to where it actually is at the time you see it. We may infer the same mechanism is at work when we consider an event that will occur at a slightly longer time in the future, such as when one puts on the brakes softly as soon as the car in front begins to slow down. One plans his/her future by extrapolating what he/she thinks might happen if things continue in a certain way. The farther one extrapolates into the future, the more errors one is likely to make.

This dt look-ahead process as performed by neuronal circuits, amazing though it may seem, is not some clever invention by the brain to be somehow better or quicker at what it already does adequately. Rather, it grows out of the tumblings of natural selection, the process that evolved the brain to operate in a predictive fashion to generate such premotor images. This is the only way the brain can keep up with what it needs to do: emulate reality as quickly and efficiently as possible, dissipatively, so that we may negotiate the external world from moment to changing moment.

But how does the brain emulate reality, and how does it generate the mindness state? We must further our understanding of how the brain generates/controls movement. It is time for us to remember our cursory discussion from chapter 1 concerning electrotonic coupling of neurons and the generation of oscillatory and resonant states; such concepts are fundamental to the understanding of the pulsatile and synergistic organization of movement.

The Discontinuous Control of Movement: Organizing the System

Let us recall chapter 1 for a moment and bring to mind the important work of Graham Brown. Brown, you will remember, viewed activities of the motor system as organized not on a reflexological basis, but rather on a self-referential basis. The reflexological view held that movement execution is (and must be) driven initially by a sensory cue arriving from the external world. Brown, by contrast, suggested that movement execution is driven initially by central neuronal circuits whose functional properties can and would generate the appropriate patterns of activity to "will" the body into organized movement. This view is referred to as self-referential because although information arising from the external world may be a sufficient reason for organized movement (behavior), such information is not necessary for its actual physiological genesis. Brown demonstrated that although sensory input is necessary for the modulation of ongoing movement, it is not required for its generation (figure 2.4). These points may be related back to the two fundamental control components of voluntary movement. The internally generated initial feedforward component does not require sensory feedback during execution. The later feedback component requires sensory input from the periphery for fine tuning a voluntary movement.

Following Brown's work, the question became one of mechanism. If not reflex/sensory input, then just what is at the heart of such central circuits that could provide the intrinsic drive to generate organized movement? Although the answers to these inquiries have been slow in coming, the self-referential approach to the organization of motor control has been given a shot in the arm by the discovery of intrinsic neuronal oscillations and the specific ionic currents necessary for their generation (Llinás 1988).

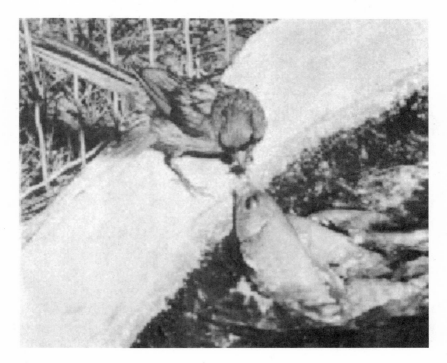

Figure 2.4
An example of a self-referential, stereotypical behavior pattern triggered in the absence of its appropriate external stimulus. In a small pond, a cardinal feeds minnows, which rose to the surface looking for food. Over several weeks the bird fed them, probably because her nest had been destroyed. Having lost her nestlings, the bird was most likely responding inappropriately to a dominant parental instinct, that is, the sight of stimuli similar to her nestling (small open mouths) elicited an inborn and stereotypic behavior (known as a "fixed action pattern," or FAP; see chapter 7). This behavior is genetically determined and presents a complex interaction with environmental stimuli. The Dutch ethologist Niko Tinbergen was one of the first to study such behaviors in vertebrates. (From N. Tinbergen, *Animal Behavior.* New York: Time Inc., 1966.)

It should be clear that oscillatory neuronal behavior relates to the organizational operation of the motor apparatus as a whole. Oscillatory behavior underlies, or at least is associated with, the generation of an overt, rhythmic activity, as we see in the movements of walking or scratching, and in involuntary rhythmic movements such as the physiological tremor. Regarding tremor and its relationship to the initiation of voluntary movement, we arrived at the understanding that this 8–12 Hz periodic activity seen in muscle represented the reflection of a supraspinal motor control system that operates in a pulsatile, discontinuous fashion. Moreover, this system is believed to synchronize the elements of the motor apparatus as a whole to facilitate the combination of the different premotor signals required for the generation of a meaningful movement (figure 2.5). It is amazing that this control system operates in a noncontinuous way when one considers that the conduction velocities (speed of nervous signaling) of the differing neuronal pathways that must exercise control over movement most likely vary widely. Because different neuronal elements (which relate to a movement) cannot be physiologically informed ahead of time of the activities simultaneously generated by other possible (neuronal) contributors to the final movement, the control system must therefore have a clock or a timing device. This device allows for certain events, correct choices, to be more likely than others. At the very core of the clock or timing device is its oscillatory, periodic behavior.

Where does such a control system reside, to synchronize motor control signals so that movement is executed in an organized, expeditious fashion? It must be centrally located (it does not reside in the muscle or spinal cord). The spinal cord is more than capable of sustaining a rhythmic movement—like the proverbial decapitated chicken!—but it does not have the wherewithal to organize and generate a directed movement on its own. Central timing must display oscillatory neuronal behavior and also oscillatory ensemble behavior (one or two neurons here and there are not enough to time the organized execution of movement); it ought also to show an overt and deep association with movement itself.

The Inferior Olive

Several groups of central neurons (nuclei) such as the inferior olivary nucleus (IO) play a fundamental role in movement coordination. In the case

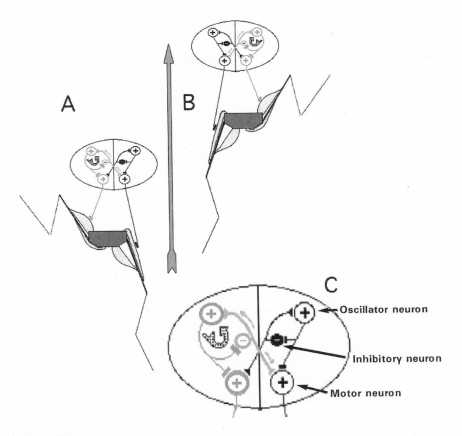

Figure 2.5
Half-paired center. Stereotypical oscillatory behavior underlying directed movement is driven by circuits such as those illustrated here. Activation of the motor neuron innervating the flexor muscle in the left limb is accompanied by the simultaneous inhibition of its counterpart in the right limb, and vice versa. This alternating paired activation/inhibition is controlled by a central pattern generator originating higher up in the neuraxis. (Drawing by R. Llinás, unpublished.)

of the IO neurons, their axons group to form nerve fiber bundles that travel together into a portion of the brain known as the cerebellum (figure 2.6). This structure is located behind the main brain mass, the cerebrum, and controls motor coordination. The fibers arising from the inferior olive end by branching on to the main neurons of the cerebellar cortex are called the Purkinje cells. These are the largest nerve cells in the brain, and the ends of the IO axons, termed climbing fibers, literally climb up over the Purkinje cells' branching dendrites (fingerlike projections providing additional surface), where neurons receive input from other neurons (figure 2.6). As mentioned earlier, most movement control processing occurs in the cerebellum, and the climbing fibers, some of the most powerful synaptic inputs in the vertebrate central nervous system, play an important role in motor control (Eccles et al. 1966), as Purkinje cells are inhibitory onto their target neurons (Ito 1984, p. 61). Damage to the IO or to the climbing fibers causes immediate, severe, and irreversible abolition of many aspects of motor coordination, both in the timing of movements and in the correct negotiation of movement through three-dimensional space: wrong timing, wrong placement. The IO plays such an important role in timing that animals with damage to this system have problems learning new motor behaviors (Welsh et al. 1995; Welsh 1998). However, this does not mean that the cerebellum is the seat of motor learning, as some contemporary scientists believe.

Axons of the IO (inferior olive) cells give rise to the cerebellar climbing fibers (figure 2.6). Intracellular recording from such cells (see chapter 4) has demonstrated that the transmembrane voltage in these cells oscillates spontaneously (at 8–12 Hz). IO cells fire action potentials (spikes) at a frequency of 1–2 Hz (spikes per second) (Llinás 1981), and although they do not fire on every oscillation, when they do, it occurs at the peak of the wave. It should be pointed out that this is not an isolated phenomenon, but that such IO activity is seen across many species.

Today, we know that IO cells fire their action potentials in a rhythmic fashion, and we also know a great deal about the intricate interplay of membrane conductances (ionic flow) that underlies the generation of this oscillatory activity. This rhythmic activity is sometimes referred to as regenerative firing, for such cells are capable of generating action potentials without the help of excitatory input converging on them (Llinás and Yarom 1981a, b).

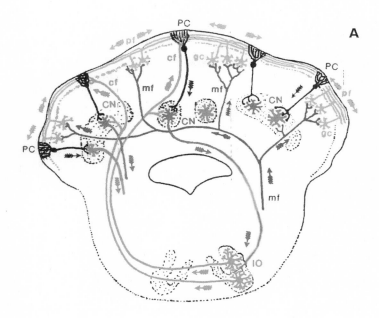

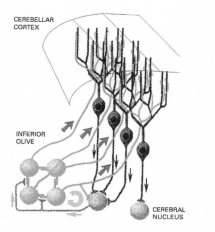

Figure 2.6
(*A*) Circuit diagram showing the connections between the inferior olive (IO), cerebellar cortex and cerebellar nuclei (CN). (Modified from Llinás 1987, figure 23.5) (*B*) Detail of the IO-cerebellum-CN loop. The climbing fiber axons of the IO terminate on the Purkinje cell, while Purkinje cell axons project to and terminate in the CN. The CN cells project their axons in turn back to the IO. (Modified from Llinás and Welsh, 1993, figure 1)

Imagine that the pattern of electrical activity occurring simultaneously in many cells that sense each other electrically is imparted to the Purkinje cells of the cerebellar cortex by the climbing fibers and to cells in the cerebellar nuclei that can drive movement (see figure 2.6, above). If we remember that the cerebellum is the neuronal area where most of the control of movement coordination is processed, then we are getting closer, physiologically speaking, to our timing signal for the control of movement. The issue here is that oscillation of the inferior olive results in a slight tremor that we all have at close to 10 Hz, even when we are not moving (Llinás et al. 1975). This slight movement (known as physiological tremor) serves to time movements, like a metronome does when we are learning to play a musical instrument. Interestingly, no one can move faster than they can tremble. Indeed, one more echo of Bernstein's words is in order: "Is there no reason to suppose that this [tremor] frequency marks the appearance of rhythmic oscillations in the excitability of all, or of the main elements of the . . . motor apparatus, in which a mutual synchronization through rhythm is doubtless necessary?" (Bernstein 1967).

We have discussed physiological tremor and have surmised that it is a reflection at the musculoskeletal level of a central timing mechanism. The studies of IO anatomy and function are all consistent with the idea that the IO is in fact operating as a timing mechanism for the rhythmic orchestration of such premotor signals required for the genesis of coordinated movement. But the proof is in the pudding: we have chased tremor up into the brain, can we chase it back down again?

As detailed in box 2.1, there is strong scientific evidence to indicate the relationship of the IO to tremor. An important question to ask is whether the IO is rhythmically active when a voluntary rhythmic movement is performed. We know that the initiation of a voluntary movement is highly associated with the phase of tremor. In one study, by use of multiple, simultaneous microelectrode recordings of Purkinje cell activity during pulsatile protrusions of the tongue in the free-moving, unanesthetized rat, a clear and robust pattern of activity of the IO was observed (Welsh 1998). These findings, which are much too involved to detail here, give significant support to the idea that the pulsate organization of movement may well be related to rhythmic, ensemble output of the IO (Smith 1998; Welsh 1998).

Box 2.1
Harmaline

A particular pharmacological agent known as harmaline, when applied directly to the IO, can enhance the membrane potential oscillations of IO neurons, locking them into a powerful, 10-Hz, synchronous discharge. When administered systematically, harmaline induces widespread rhythmic activation of muscles throughout the body; this is observed behaviorally as a strong and highly stereotypic 10-Hz tremor (Villablanca and Riobo 1970; Lamarre et al. 1971; de Montigny and Lamarre 1973). Furthermore, when set up for intracellular recording as well, this preparation revealed that the highly repetitive and rhythmic activity of single olivary cells, reflected at the Purkinje cell level, was tightly time-locked to the 10-Hz tremor and remained so through long-term recording (figure 2.7) (Llinás and Volkind 1973; Llinás 1981). Upon experimental destruction of the IO, regardless of the presence of harmaline, the behavioral tremor was abolished (Llinás et al. 1975).

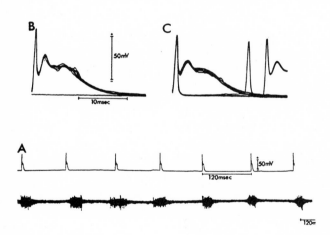

Figure 2.7
Either systemic or localized application of harmaline induces the IO to generate a 10-Hz synchronous discharge. See text for details.

About Motor Control: Principles and Ideas

We have spent a good deal of time and focus on the issue of motor control. At this point, it may seem that we have drifted quite far from our expedition into how the mind arose from evolution, but we are actually much closer. Before we move onward, let us recapitulate what we have learned about how the brain controls movement. We will need these ideas and principles as we press toward the evolutionary/physiological infrastructure of the mind. *The brain's control of organized movement gave birth to the generation and nature of the mind.*

Continuous-through-time control of movement, combined with simultaneous but independent control of individual muscles, leads to a physiologically untenable functional overhead for the brain, even if all neurons contained within it were used, which they are not. Most motor processing is handled by the cerebellum and its associated incoming and outgoing systems. Motor control therefore must operate as a process whereby motor output is restricted (controlled) to an optimally small subset of all possible movements. Clearly such optimization must be born out of principles of neural function that simplify the enormity of the underlying computation.

Heuristically speaking, this optimization/simplification process would be discontinuous through time and the target of such pulsatile control would be functional collectives of muscles, synergies "expected" or predisposed to work together for a given aspect of a movement sequence. This control, which is necessarily pulsatile, must operate often enough to minimize accelerative transients so that jerkiness in a movement is smoothed out. Finally, this control must be labile. It must be able to reconfigure itself readily, allowing for a nearly infinite ability to appropriate need-to-use-this-moment-only combinations and recombinations of muscle synergies. The ability of this control system to do so should mirror in time the transience of muscle configurations as they are recruited and discarded during a voluntary movement sequence.

From a physiological standpoint, we see thorough and quite convincing evidence that the olivocerebellar system is the prime candidate for a neural assembly capable of optimizing and simplifying motor control: it is temporally pulsatile and rapidly, dynamically self-reorganizing in the spatial domain.

It is clear that prediction is possible when well-defined segments of time can be calculated. These small fragments of time must be well defined so that they may be properly operated on, properly controlled if you will. A well-behaved oscillatory movement can be well controlled because one generates movement at short time steps. One does not invest more than a certain amount of movement when one is not certain. This is called moving cautiously or tentatively. Such a movement strategy is not always conducive to survival. A boxer can deliver a punch in 100 milliseconds. If you don't see the punch coming you will not be able to dodge it (tentative dodging is not an alternative). So what does "see it coming" mean? You must know that if the shoulder is moving forward, a punch may follow 200 milliseconds later. Boxing requires rapid prediction and rapid execution, a bit like playing the stock market. They are both excellent examples of the need for prediction based on information input and of coordinated execution requiring temporal coherence in neuronal activity. But all of this is important even when reaching for a carton of milk in the refrigerator. We know because often we misjudge the carton's weight and hit the upper shelf!

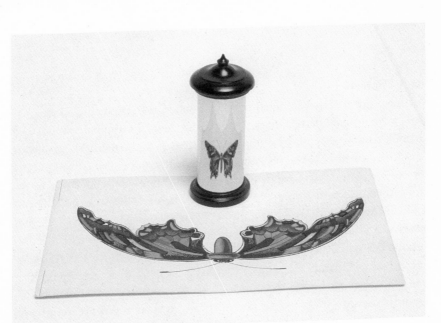

Anamorphic picture of a butterfly with catoptic cone, c. 1848. Science Museum/
Science & Society Picture Library, London

3

The Embedding of Universals through the Embedding of Motricity

A Synthesis of Mind

It is fair to say that present-day science can be characterized by a stronger tendency toward isolated analysis than synthesis. The study of neuroscience is no exception; our research often fails to reach past the objective description of the properties of neurons and of the networks they weave. For those of us who believe in the necessity of a seamless, contextual continuum of analysis from the molecular to the psychophysical level, it is heartening to note that this global approach has been implemented in certain areas, most particularly in the study of sensory systems.

In the visual system for example, it is generally agreed that by transforming lightwave fronts into images, the geometric and refractive properties of the eye provide the context for the organization of the visual system at all levels of evolution. This trend toward a unifying synthesis is also reflected in our thinking about other sensory organs. The accepted view today is that the resonant properties of the basilar membrane in the cochlear organ of Corti in the inner ear (figure 3.1) and the spatial arrangement of the semicircular canals of the vestibular organ provide the necessary coordinate systems for the neural representation of sound and angular acceleration of the head, respectively. However, as we move

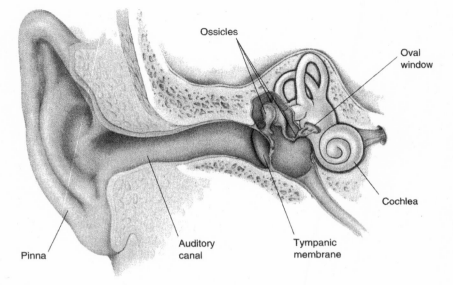

Figure 3.1
Diagram of the auditory system, including the outer, middle, and inner ear, containing the cochlear organ of Corti. See text for other details. (From Bear et al. 1996, figure 11.3)

away from the peripheral sensory systems, it becomes increasingly difficult to keep a clear focus on the overall context into which each level of analysis must ultimately be woven. And so, in this chapter it is my aim to attempt a context-dependent analysis and to explain how the brain's ability to understand is intimately related to the evolution of its organizational structure.

From chapters 1 and 2, we saw that for any actively moving creature, predictive ability, and therefore a central nervous system, is indispensable. Such creatures must have a robust strategy for internally referencing the consequences of their comings and goings in a world ruled by simple yet relentless natural selection. This referencing or understanding of the external world comes about through the functional juxtaposing of internally generated sensorimotor images with the sensory-referred properties, or "universals" present in the world outside. In chapter 2, we considered that the generation of sensorimotor images occurs through the intrinsic properties of the brain and that such properties are in every way similar to those that rapidly construct and employ muscle synergies for movement execution. Such premotor constructs, fleetingly gathered and dissolved functional patterns of neuronal activity, must emulate external reality in order to determine the consequences of their movements. The properties of this external world, universals, must somehow be embedded into the functional workings or neuronal circuitry of the brain. Such internalization, the embedding of universals into an internal functional space, is one of the essentials of brain function.

Can we describe such complex and fleeting entities from a physiological point of view? Yes, and we shall do so later in this chapter; at this point we shall begin the process by referring to the functional geometry of the brain.

The brain does not actually compute anything, not in the sense of the algorithmic handling of ones and zeros that characterizes Alan Turing's digital "universal computer" (Turing 1947; Millican and Clark 1996). Our reality emulator acts primarily as the prerequisite for coordinated, directed motricity; it does so by generating a predictive image of an event to come that causes the creature to react or behave accordingly. Such an image may be considered a premotor template that serves as a planning platform for behavior or purposeful action. It may also be considered as the basis from which consciousness, in all living forms, is generated.

The brain did not just pop into existence out of nowhere, without any evolutionary trace, so it is probable that it already possesses at birth as much of an a priori order to its intricate organization as does the rest of the body. All the bones, joints, and muscles, and most of what they are capable of doing, are in principle already inscribed in the geometry of the system when we are born. We also possess at birth the quality of plasticity, the ability to adapt to the changing circumstances of the world we live in by changing those biological parameters that have been predesigned to be malleable. Human language is a good example. We hone our ability to recognize inherently human phonemes by discarding those we do not hear during our developing years (Kuhl et al. 1997; Kuhl 2000). In this process, we enhance our ability to acquire one human language as opposed to another. But we must keep in mind that plasticity can occur only within clearly defined constraints. As we saw in chapter 2, regardless of training or personal effort we cannot make movements much faster than

10 Hz (Llinás 1991). We can greatly increase muscle mass with specific exercise, but we cannot alter the number of individual muscle fibers in the body, only their mass, and even that has an upper limit. One can apply this rule to the brain as well: the intrinsic organization of nervous systems can be enriched through plasticity and learning, but only up to a predetermined point.

One may then ask, if the perceptual properties of the brain are not learned *de novo,* where and how do they originate? Well, they must arise through evolution, of course. We can actually observe in detail these innate capabilities of nervous system function if, for instance, we look at the visual system at birth. From the first moment that light hits the retina, the ability to assign some meaning to visual images is present in most animals, including primates (Wiesel and Hubel 1974; Sherk and Stryker 1976; Ramachandran et al. 1977; Hubel and Wiesel 1979). This brings us to the concept of a neurological a priori. The foundation concept itself is by no means new, as it has been a philosophical issue since the days of Immanuel Kant (Kant 1781). The only difference today is that by virtue of what we understand of the functional properties of nerve cells and the brain, we may move the issue of a neurological a priori from one solely of epistemological concern to that of a developmental, phylogenetic concern.

Before we head into the deeper questions of how the brain came to use predictive, sensorimotor representations, and then to extract and embed a set of universals that may represent the external world, I must bring up the issue of the brain as a closed system modulated by the senses. An open system, if you will recall, is one that accepts inputs from the environment, processes them, and returns them to the world reflexively regardless of their complexity.

A logical extension of this view is that the central nervous system could be initially in a close to *tabula rasa* configuration at birth. If so, it should be fundamentally a learning machine. This view is still pervasive and is supported mostly by a branch of science known as neural networks. It has also given tremendous impetus to the electronics industry because the practical results are very real and add an important control technique. However, this approach, while useful in other applications, explains very little concerning the actual functioning of the nervous system itself and, moreover, has no reply to the observation that there are clear areas of invariance in nervous system function among species. On this latter point, neurobiology and neuroscience hold that a basic similarity of phenotype (observable physical traits) within species and even among species is related to similar neuronal function. Thus these disciplines assume that to a large extent brain structure is under the control of genetic determinism—far removed from the tabula rasa idea.

The closed-system hypothesis (Llinás 1974, 1987), on the other hand, argues for a primarily self-activating system, one whose organization is geared toward the generation of intrinsic images. We saw in chapter 2 that given the nature of the thalamocortical system, sensory input from the external world only gains significance via the preexisting functional disposition of the brain at that moment, its internal context. It follows that such a self-activating system is capable of emulating reality (generating emulative representations or images) even in the absence of input from such reality, as occurs in dream states or daydreaming (which we shall discuss in later chapters). From this one may draw a very important conclusion. This intrinsic order of function represents the fundamental, core activity of the brain. This core activity may be modified (to a point!) through sensory experience and through the effects of motor activity, the latter in response to the external world or to internally generated images or concepts. We may view emotions in this light as excellent examples of internally generated intrinsic events and as such, they are also excellent examples of premotor templates in primitive forms. Such templates are also evident in higher vertebrates, if the motor suppression that often constrains the behavioral manifestation of emotion is also considered part of the motor realm, as in "curb your anger!" These issues will be handled more thoroughly in ensuing chapters, mainly chapter eight.

To return to our hypothesis: as a closed system, the central nervous system must have developed over evolutionary time as a neuronal network that initially handled very simple connectivity relations between sensory and motor systems. As the nervous system evolved, the constraints generated by the coordinate systems that describe the body were slowly embedded into a functional space within the nervous system. This provided a natural, activity dependent understanding that a creature would have of its own body, an easily agreed upon prerequisite for purposeful movement (as in the play behavior displayed by most young animals, really an exploration of the properties of internal functional space). Furthermore, as with those genetically selected-for aspects of the body, such embedding of coordinate systems into a functional space within the nervous system slowly became genetically determined as well (Pellionisz and Llinás 1982). And so we see, following straight Darwinism, that a neurological a priori was developed over the hundreds of millions of years of vertebrate and invertebrate phylogeny. From this comes the global message of the first section of this book: that we may consider cognition to be not only a functional state, but an intrinsic property of the brain and a neurological a priori, as well. The ability to cognate does not have to be learned; only the particular content of cognition as it specifically relates to the particulars around us must be learned.

The Embedding of Single Cell Motricity to Form a System

Let us now turn to an examination of how the brain came to embed the properties of the external world, how it carries this out, and the evolutionary relationship of this phenomenon to the generation of such an amazing functional space as mindness.

Let us begin with some general thoughts on how our brain negotiates the immense differences between the properties of the external world and a neuronally generated representation of those properties. Suppose you wish to draw the face of someone you once knew, and you are conveniently able to draw quite well. Consider the numerous input/output brain events that must be involved in successfully carrying out this desired task. With delicately executed movements, you must reproduce—externalize—your internal image of that person, an image that was formed by your brain from sensory inputs arising from the external world. What is the nature of the functional space we have referred to that allows the brain to construct and evaluate such an internal image and then to externalize it? It is not difficult to understand that the externalization of any internal image can only be carried out through movement: drawing, speaking, gesturing with one's arms. What I must stress here is that the brain's understanding of anything, whether factual or abstract, arises from our manipulations of the external world, by our moving within the world and thus from our sensory-derived experience of it. I should like to propose how, from the electrotonic and oscillatory coupling concepts we have discussed at length, the internalization process, the "embedding," could have occurred.

A good preliminary example: how did the heart evolve? The answer, although not at first obvious, is really quite simple. It evolved through the process of organizing single-cell motricity so that macroscopic motricity came about. In mechanistic terms it meant coordinating the bioelectric properties of single cells so that they added together to generate a "system."

Single-cell motricity is derived from the activation of contractile machinery often rhythmically modulated by intrinsic voltage oscillations of the cell's surface membrane driven by transmembrane ionic concentration differences. Experimentally, we can grow individual cardiac cells in a dish, and they will beat on their own (for reviews, see DeHaan and Sacks 1972; Mitcheson et al. 1998). Once these single cardiac cells come into contact with each other, they become electrotonically coupled, one cell to the next, whereupon they begin to beat together. What one sees at this stage are waves of contraction, driven and determined by impedance-matched connectivity. As this sheath proceeds to fold on itself and make pockets, or heart chambers, the contractility is not equally distributed (isotropic) in space. Rather than simple contraction waves, the added geometry of a pocket transforms a contracting cellular sheath into a pump. And so single-cell motricity and its intrinsic oscillatory properties have generated, through specific topological reorganization, a macroscopic event by the coupling of such properties through connectivity. This is the basis of movement of all types, and will permeate our discussion: *the organization and function of our brains are based on the embedding of motricity over evolution* (cf. Llinás 1986).

From Contractile Muscle Tissue to the Organization of Brain

Let us consider a beautifully illustrative case of the general organization of brain development, that of the elasmobranchs (sharks). The embryo of these sharks develops in an egg case that allows oxygen through. In order for oxygen to be distributed appropriately throughout the tissues of the

developing embryo, there must be a continuous movement of the fluid inside the egg (ooplasm), and so the embryo undulates rhythmically, in a sinusoidal fashion. Now here we have a very significant point, for at this
stage of development, the movement is not generated by nervous system
activity (Harris and Whiting 1954). In fact, the muscle cells comprising
the musculature that generates this rhythmic movement have yet to be
innervated by their respective motoneurons! How then are the muscles
operative? At this stage of development, the muscle cells are all electrically coupled (Blackshaw and Warner 1976; Kahn et al. 1982; Armstrong et al. 1983). It is very similar to the heart example above, except
that this is not a heart—this is an animal. Being coupled in this fashion,
the electrical signal that causes contraction of one muscle cell spreads
rapidly from cell to cell; thus it sets up the rhythmic undulations seen at
the whole animal level. Because this movement is born purely from the
muscle cells themselves, this event is referred to as the "myogenic" stage
of motricity (Harris and Whiting 1954). This myogenic stage of motricity
serves many important physiological functions; for one, it begins the organization of the creature's eventual direction of forward movement in
the ocean.

In the next stage of development a very significant functional transformation occurs. The spinal cord starts putting out the axons of the motor
neurons that travel or "migrate" to their target muscles. At this point, the
motor neurons are also electrotonically coupled (O'Donovan 1987;
Walton and Navarrete 1991; Mazza et al. 1992; Kandler and Katz 1995).
As the growing axons begin to contact and innervate their target muscle
cells, forming electrochemical synapses (that we spoke of in chapter 2),
the muscle cells cease being electrotonically coupled (Armstrong et al.
1983); this is the end of the so-called myogenically derived motricity.
What we see is that the ability to make undulatory movements has been
displaced from the muscle cells to the interior of the spinal cord (figure
3.2). In other words, the motility properties of the muscular mass have
been embedded into the connectivity and intrinsic electrical properties of
the spinal cord neuronal circuits. This is now the stage known as
neurogenic motricity.

Thus, there is a close impedance matching (having the same dynamic
properties) of neurogenic movement to the properties of the muscle. The

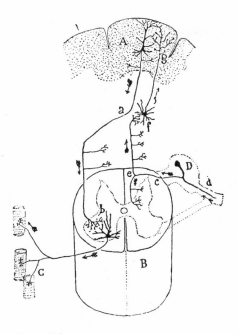

Figure 3.2
Diagram of the central pathways for somatosensory input and voluntary motor excitation from the cerebral cortex. (*A*) Cerebral cortex. (*B*) Spinal cord. (*C*) Muscle fibers receiving input from spinal cord motor neurons. (*D*) Afferent fibers from the periphery via the dorsal root ganglion. (From Ramón y Cajal, 1911, figure 27).

upshot of this is that the external properties of the animal have begun to be internalized in the brain. The motoneurons stay electrotonically coupled until the upper part of the system, the brain stem (also at this point electrotonically coupled), starts making its synaptic connections with the motor neurons (Armstrong et al. 1983; Bleasel and Pettigrew 1992; Welsh and Llinás 1997; Chang et al. 2000). At that point, the motor neurons become electrotonically decoupled, but the upper part of the system remains coupled. In addition to becoming electrotonically decoupled at this stage of development, motor neurons also begin to receive synaptic inputs from other parts of the nervous system that do not specifically relate to the activation of given muscle groups. These additional inputs relate more to the global movement of the total mass of the animal, and involve the vestibular system, the organ of equilibrium that informs the motor neuronal network (thus the musculoskeletal system) about holistic properties of motricity. Am I swimming right side up, or upside-down? It helps the animal organize its motricity with respect to a larger frame of reference than its own body, such as the gravitational pull of the Earth and the inertial consequences of movement at right angles to gravitation—to "think" left and right, and up and down. Then encephalization appears (the formation of the mature aspects of the brain, its shape, and its connectivity). Animals that are elongated tend to move along the path of least resistance, in the direction of their long axis. This in turn stages the direction of most common movement, let's call it forward, and it is the forward end through which the creature will encounter whatever is new in its environment more often than the other extreme (which tends to be naturally selected out, for obvious reasons). It follows that here at the front end is the smartest place to put the telereceptive sensory systems such as olfaction and sight. Here at the leading end will also be the jaws, and here a head develops with a brain, protected by exoskeleton, the skull, which fortuitously serves, among other things, as a bumper. By the same token, the unwanted products of digestion are expelled out the back end, hopefully never to be encountered again.

The Internalization of the Body Plant

And so we see that the property of motricity is being internalized—the beast is literally pulling itself up by its bootstraps! It is the only way to explain the incorporation of external motricity inside. The only way is by pulling it in upwards; the system takes properties from the outside and pulls them immediately inside. Through intrinsic oscillatory properties and electrical coupling, these properties are pulled up the neuraxis and into the encephalization of the brain. So what do we have? The ability to think, which arises from the internalization of movement. This was proposed in chapter 1 when I mentioned that thinking was a central event born out of an increasing number of successful possible motor strategies. The issue is that thinking ultimately represents movement, not just of body parts or of objects in the external world, but of perceptions and complex ideas as well.

How is this embedding of motricity actually accomplished and why should we want to know? Perhaps in understanding how this was/is accomplished, we will understand something about our very own nature, as the mechanism for internalization must be very closely related to how we process our own thinking, and to the nature of mind and of learning by experience. The short answer to the question, as we have just discussed, is that we do this by the activation and transfer of intrinsic, oscillatory electrical properties. Basically, motor neurons fire intrinsically, muscles contract rhythmically, and the receptors in muscles and joints respond to the movement and inform motor neurons about their success in producing movement and the direction of such movement in body coordinates. In other words, when I activate motor neurons, I get a sensory echo—and the echo somehow seems to be related to my body's response to the motor order. In fact, during development, embryos generate continuous bouts of muscle tremor not unlike small epileptic fits (Hamburger and Balaban 1963; Bekoff et al. 1975). This is more than a metaphor; epileptic activity may in fact be among the most primitive of all functional states, given that it is so very similar across differing species and different people, and independent of social and environmental factors. It is a bit like coughing or sneezing in this regard.

Cephalization

This upward march of cephalization is seen not only in embryonic development (ontogeny), but also (and much more slowly) in phylogenetic development. For instance, the phylogenetic stage of the adult lamprey is the stage of neurogenic motricity in which motor neurons are still electrically coupled (Ringham 1975; Christensen 1976; Shapovalov 1977; Batueva and Shapovalov 1977; Batueva 1987). And so, in lampreys, as in the case of the heart, motricity (swimming for them) has to do with intrinsic neuronal activity and with how these neurons are electrically coupled with each other. This moving forward or backward may be thought of as equivalent to a set of heartbeats. The difference is that the animal moves front to back, and it is not the muscles but rather the neurons driving the muscles that are electrically coupled. The neurons move the muscles, and the muscles return a message to the neurons about the outside world by taking into consideration—simply experiencing—the unevenness of the terrain the animal is moving in or on. For example, the changing currents it swims through or the bottom it crawls over.

This brings up an important, rather critical evolutionary point. The advantage of separating the movement generating property from the movement pattern generator is that specialized pattern generators (motor neurons and their connectivity) can produce, by combinatorial properties among themselves, far more complex types of motricity. For example, leaving the issue of walking to the intrinsic properties of muscles themselves will not get us very far down the sidewalk. To walk, we need the intrinsic properties of the neuronal circuitry of the spinal cord (and farther up the neuraxis toward the head, as we saw in chapter 2, for its initiation) to generate the coordinated, rhythmic drive to the appropriate, alternating muscle synergies involved in gait. Similarly, although the heart will beat rhythmically on its own, it is the brainstem that modulates up or down the periodicity of the intrinsic rhythm.

Internal Functional Space: The External World and the Internal World Have Different Coordinate System Reference Frames

Now the reader should have a grasp of how evolution has employed cell-biological rules to embed properties of the external world into the very nature of nervous system organizational structure. The next step is to examine how this embedding process is recapitulated in nervous system function. I began this chapter by pointing out that perhaps the most important issue in brain research today is that of the internalization or embedding of the universals of the external world into an internal functional space. Let me now address what an internal functional space is and how it must work, given that the brain operates as a closed system.

It should be understood now that for an organism to successfully negotiate the external world, the nervous system must be able to handle expeditiously (process and understand) the universals of this external world arriving via sensory input. The processed information must be converted subsequently into well-executed motor output delivered back into the external world. This conceptually, but not physiologically, amorphous area of transformation between sensory input and motor output is what is meant by an internal functional space. It is clear that the properties of this space and the properties of the external world are not the same; and yet, for motor output to have usefully expressed meaning, there must be a continuity of similarity. This internal functional space that is made up of neurons must represent the properties of the external world—it must somehow be homomorphic with it. Just as a translator must operate with conceptual continuity between the two different languages he/she is translating, so too must this internal functional space preserve conceptual continuity.

How then does this internal functional space operate? Well, we must ask what the translational—indeed transformational—properties of this space need to subserve in order to provide this homomorphic continuity between the sensory-derived properties of the external world and subsequent motor output. It is a serious question of the differences in coordinate system reference frames between the external and internal worlds and how continuity between perception and execution may/must exist. A. Pellionisz and I addressed these questions in a series of papers spanning well over a decade of research (see, for example, Pellionisz and Llinás 1979, 1980, 1982, 1985).

A helpful example, at the intuitive level, that sensorimotor transformation truly is coordinate system independent, would be the following. Let us return to our drawing example from the beginning of this chapter (p. 58), but this time you draw two versions of the face of the person you once knew. The first version is a large drawing, using mainly your shoulder and elbow joints and an appropriately large drawing charcoal (figure 3.3 A, left). For the second version, you draw the face with your forearm held rigid and you only use finger movements to generate the drawing (figure 3.3A, right). Obviously, this drawing will be much smaller. If we then photographically compensate for size (figure 3.3 B) and superimpose the two pictures (figure 3.3 C), the two faces will be remarkably similar (if of course you can draw well! The drawing shown in figure 3.3 was made by a well-known artist). What does this say? It says that the internal representation of the face can be externalized using entirely different sensory and motor coordinate systems—that the internal vector

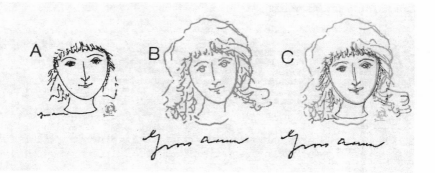

Figure 3.3
Externalization using different sets of motor and sensory coordinates. (*A*) Composite showing a large drawing made by the artist Arnold Gross of Budapest when allowing full movement of his elbow and shoulder, and a small version of the same drawing made when he restricted movement to the hand alone (*bottom right*). (*B*) Enlargement of the small drawing in (*A*). (*C*) Superimposition of (*A*) and (*B*) showing the great similarity between the two drawings. (From Llinás, 1987, figure 23.6, p. 355).

representing the face may be transformed into a motor-execution space in a fashion independent of the coordinate-system. This is a clear example of the fact that tensorial properties of the brain operate in sensorimotor transformations.

Functional Geometry

A second organizing principle may be equally important—one that is based on temporal rather than spatial relationships among neurons. This temporal mapping may be viewed as a type of functional geometry (Pellionisz and Llinás 1982). This mechanism has been difficult to study until recently because it requires the simultaneous measurement of activity from large numbers of neurons and is not a parameter usually considered in neuroscience. The central tenet of the temporal mapping hypothesis can be summarized simply. Spatial mapping creates a finite universe of possible representations. Adding the component of time to the spatial mapping generates an immensely larger set of possible representations as categorization is achieved by the superposition of spatial and temporal mapping via thalamocortical resonant iteration. It is the temperospatial dialogue between the thalamus and the cortex that generates subjectivity.

The case of the CNS (central nervous system) is comparable to taking a picture of a moving object, not with an instantaneous flash, but replacing the light with a set of lights (in the CNS, axons), each having a different conduction time. Creating an internal "picture" of the external reality in the CNS in such a manner, through differently delayed neuronal signals, means that simultaneous external events will not be represented in the CNS as simultaneous. Conversely, simultaneous onset of firing of a group of neurons with different conduction velocities will not produce a set of simultaneous external events, either. "Simultaneous occurrence" can be detected by a clock only where an instantaneous (or otherwise synchronous) access is available to it from the "timed" events. Because in the CNS the difference between the speed of the controlled events (e.g., movements) and that of the controller signals (slowly propagating neuronal firings) is not great enough to allow for instantaneous and synchronous access to a clock through the axons, simultaneity cannot be established. Therefore, this concept is not applicable to the internal functioning of neuronal systems. (To give a vivid example of the problem of space-timing by a central clock, consider an attempt to coordinate the position of speeding battle tanks from military headquarters, not with instantaneous radio signals, but by cavalry messengers).

It is clear that if no superfast command signal is available, an alternative mode of space-timing must be found that does not rely on the concept of simultaneity. In the same vein, because simultaneity of events within the CNS could not be established by the use of any "brain clock," even if such a device were to exist, then the brain must be using an alternative mode of space-timing.

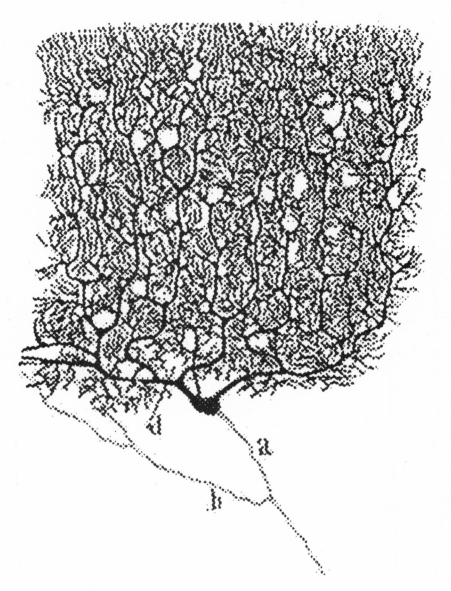

Picture of a typical neuron.

4

Nerve Cells and Their Personalities

Single Cells Give Rise to Single Minds

As mindness is one of many global functional states generated by the brain, we may also then say that mindness is one of many states generated by a society of neurons. We have reviewed the concept of mindness, and how its acquisition was driven by the evolutionary embedding of motricity. Using principles underlying the long-accepted disciplines of electrophysiology and biophysics, let us now ground these views in firm science.

To address issues concerning the workings of the mind, we can describe the cell-biological rules that evolution must have employed to produce the nervous system, namely the evolutionary trial and error approach of natural selection, at both the single cell and whole animal level.

One must first identify the property of nerve cells that allows them to be organized into the networked society capable of representing universals and their meaningful interaction with the outside world in real time. This property is electrical activity at the microscopic level, the electrical properties of neurons provided by their intrinsic electrical excitability, their synaptic connectivity, and the architecture of the networks they weave. The macroscopic architecture can be easily understood. For example, consider that the interconnected neurons in the retina must form a thin layer of transparent tissue spread across the black inner surface of the eye cup so that the lenses at the front of the eye can project a light image onto its surface. The elements that bring about this connectivity must insure that the retina transmits by electrical means a meaningful representation of the image to the brain.

It is the difference in the electrical properties and connectivity of neurons that allows networks to internalize the external world images into our brain and to transform such images into motor behavior. Such networks also generate the rapidly moving electrical storms that represent, internally, the fast and ever-changing external reality. These dissipative electrical events of the brain, rich enough to represent all that we can observe or imagine, constitute the mind. These electrical events in our networks constitute "us."

Those of us who do electrophysiological recording routinely will argue that there are few events as wondrous and exciting as listening to the sound of a live neuron speaking its own particular language and seeing this language as bursting electrical patterns flickering across the oscilloscope screen. Such intracellular recording techniques can also tell us what electrical patterns of activity are coming into a neuron from other neurons (box 4.1) When I speak of the varying electrical properties of individual neurons, this is one of the ways that we have to characterize those properties. There are other electrophysiological techniques, such as extracellular recording of electrical potentials and patch clamping membranes (high-resistance seals between the electrode and membrane surface to record the movement of tiny currents carried by ions through

Box 4.1
How Does One Study the Electrical Activity of Single Cells?

When one studies the intrinsic electrical properties of nerve cells, let's say those of the inferior olive, we see that these cells demonstrate a tuning fork-like oscillatory rhythmicity in their membrane potential. The frequency of this electrical oscillation ranges from 4–12 Hz, or 4–12 oscillations per second when recorded in vitro (Llinás and Yarom 1981a, b). The evidence of such electrical properties comes from direct recordings obtained from the interior of individual neurons by means of a microelectrode.

Intracellular recording microelectrodes are glass tubes of 1–1.5 millimeter diameter, filled with conductive fluid, the microelectrode's fine, sharpened tips can penetrate the membrane of a single cell with sometimes minimal damage to cell function. Microelectrodes are fashioned from melting and pulling very thin micropipettes. Mechanical tension is applied using a type of microrack that clamps onto and simultaneously pulls both ends of the micropipette with equal force in opposite directions; the middle of this tug-o-war is heated by an electric filament. As the glass melts, the tension causes the pipette to stretch. When it is pulled to a thin thread, the glass separates in the middle, and we now have the beginnings of two microelectrodes. After stretching, the tip of each microelectrode remains patent, and the diameter of the opening can be as small as one-fiftieth of a micron—less than one-thousandth the width of a human hair, and not visible to the naked eye.

After pulling, the electrode is back-filled with an ionic solution from a syringe to provide an electrically conducting medium. The microelectrode is then fixed to a mechanical manipulator that very precisely controls an impaling movement (a micrometer screw), which allows the microelectrode to harpoon single cells. A wire, usually silver, is inserted into this medium-filled electrode from the back end. The wire is attached, via connectors, to a very sensitive amplifier. The output signal from the amplifier is filtered and further amplified, and the signal is then digitized and stored on computer, as well as displayed on an oscilloscope. The signal is often also sent to a loudspeaker so that one may "hear" each electrical event.

The small diameter of the electrode tip makes the microelectrodes very sharp. This is important, for when the electrode tip penetrates the thin membrane of a neuron it is critical not to tear the membrane. If the membrane is torn, the delicately balanced ionic solution will be immediately altered, as the extracellular fluid—the ionic solution outside a neuron—will be in direct continuity with the cell's intracellular fluid. This severely compromises the fragile electrochemical environment inside the cell—if not killing the cell altogether.

I will not detail a tedious description of exactly how the electrode tip is successfully coaxed to impale the cell membrane of a neuron (whose cell body diameter is typically on the order of 20 microns) that resides in a particular nucleus in a particular region of the brain. One is aided by the voltage deflections on the oscilloscope, which are used as a compass to determine where the tip of the electrode is, and where it is going. Suffice it to say that the job of impaling such neurons, and the subsequent effort involved in monitoring and recording their electrical activity, is no small feat, but requires as much patience and diligence as tirelessly searching for a particular piece of straw in a barn.

individual ion channels spanning the membrane); we shall discuss them as needed. Single-cell recordings are routinely obtained from the brains of animals or humans (during neurosurgery) and can give important clues to brain function and to the diagnosing of neurological diseases. Recordings can also be obtained from tissue slices kept alive in oxygenated ionic solutions or in cultured cells in vitro.

Why Study Cells?—The Unlikeliness of Organized, Multicellular Life

It is the present view of geologists that the Earth is approximately 4.5 billion years old. Paleobiologists estimate that probably 400–500 million years after this, the first life as we know it arose, either from extraterrestrial seeding (transferring the process to another location) or by a sort of protracted spontaneous generation from assemblages of organic polymers in the inanimate ooze (Margulis and Sagan 1985). It also appears that life may have started shortly after the Earth cooled. These primordial life forms, called "prokaryotes," were essentially single-celled organisms related to the bacteria and bacteria-like organisms we know today. Prokaryotes are believed to have changed very little from these original strains; therefore they are said to have been "highly conserved" over evolution. A good example is *Escherichia coli* (figure 4.1, left), which benignly inhabits our intestines. The carcasses of *E. coli* comprise much of the solid waste that we excrete. In other parts of the body these bacteria are far from benign and can cause serious infection.

These early living organisms are essentially small compartments or bags covered by two or three types of layers. The innermost is a membrane, a thin fatty wrapping known as a lipid bilayer (double layer). External to this is generally a protective outer proteoglycan cell wall, which is sometimes covered by a third covering external to the cell wall, called a capsule (Margulis and Sagan 1985; Margulis and Olendzenski 1992; Cole et al. 1992; Lengeler et al. 1999). Inside this bag is the internal fluid or cytoplasm. Scattered within this fluid are found DNA, RNA, ribosomes, and the necessary enzymatic machinery to read evolution's genetic code and to make the proteins necessary for cellular function. Prokaryotes, however, do not separate the genetic material into a nucleus as do the more modern eukaryotic cells ("true cells").

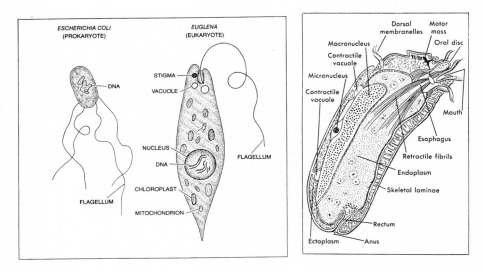

Figure 4.1
Examples of prokaryotic (*left*) and eukaryotic (*middle, right*) unicellular
lifeforms. (*Left*) *E. coli.* (*Middle*) *Euglena,* typical unspecialized protist, showing
a nucleus, mitochondria, and choloroplasts. (*Right*) *Epidinium,* a single cell
showing extensive specialization with a permanent mouth structure and digestive
system including esophagus, rectum, and anus. Retractile muscle-like fibers move
the mouth and esophagus, under control of a nerve-like network. Organs of locomotion are also controlled by a nerve-like network. These fibers all converge and
connect in a single motor mass, similar to a command center or central pattern
generator. (Left and middle figures from Gould and Gould, 1989, p. 10; right
figure from Simpson et al., 1957, figure 3-13, p. 54.)

Over the next 600 million years or so, some of these prokaryotes
learned initially to parasitize others, eventually conjoining with other
prokaryotes in a mutually beneficial manner. This is the biological meaning of the term "symbiosis." Over time, prokaryotic symbiosis led to the
formation of more elaborate single cell types; this process in evolution
probably gave rise to the first eukaryotic cell (see, for example,
Margulis and Olendzenski 1992; Ridley 1996). Eukaryotic cells are
larger than prokaryotic cells, have a well-defined outer membrane and a
richer internal architecture with membrane surrounded compartments
such as the nucleus, and well-defined small internal organs, the organelles
(figure 4.1, middle, right). As is the case with prokaryotes, eukaryotes

internally manufacture proteins that the cell needs to survive. Some of these manufactured proteins are specialized to perforate and embed themselves in the outer cell membrane. These proteins function to regulate the exchange of materials in and out of the cell, as well as to signal the regulation of many self-specific events within the cell.

So we have little islands of life contained inherently within "walls," the cellular membranes of lipid, and they are for the most part closed to the external world. One may also consider these compartments of life as closed systems in that they only communicate—and can only communicate—with the outside world by way of specialized, transmembrane gates. These are composed mostly of one or more long amino acid chains folded in complicated yet orderly tangles. By embedding themselves in and across the lipid membrane these proteins function as signaling systems that serve as specific receptors, ion channels, or pumps. These primordial compartments of life make up all life as we know it. The operation of closed systems began a long time ago; life is compartments, as is the mind.

It is illuminating that once these single-celled eukaryotic organisms first appeared, evolution took a further 2 billion years to join them into cooperating colonies of cells and what we would call the first multicellular life forms (for general references, see Margulis and Olendzenski 1992; Ridley 1996). It seems as though these eukaryotic cells had chosen not to make closely aggregated cellular societies. Two billion years is a very long period of time, particularly when one considers that once nature succeeded in making the first simple "animal," the rest of the entire animal kingdom emerged (to the present day) within 700 or so million years!

What Took So Long?

Why such an inordinate amount of time for life to move from single-celled to multicellular forms? Well, we must look at what it means for nature to actually make an "animal," a highly organized society of cells. Indeed, we must look at what is required for any successful society. There must be an agreed commonality and communication among the participants and a set of global rules that are adhered to by at least the majority of the participants. And here is the key to the mystery: evolution found that the task of imbuing single cells with the ability to communicate with one another to exchange information in a biologically meaningful manner was far more complicated than making the first single-celled life!

Although we are not really in a position to judge, still, 2 billion years does seem like a very, very long time for evolution to invent cell-to-cell communication, and we can only speculate on the reasons why. Perhaps the answer is that before certain specializations, cell aggregation simply did not provide any survival advantage: a bit selfish, but perhaps profoundly true. But when the transition from single-cell life to a multicellular society—an animal—occurred, a completely new approach to life evolved that has been with us ever since.

This approach is one that stresses total commitment to a cellular society (the "group" as self) as opposed to a total commitment to the single cell (the "individual" as self). When an animal finally evolved, true programmed "corporate death" was created. Although single-cell organisms can certainly be destroyed, we may toy with the thought that they do not normally "die" per se, but just divide. Any amoeba alive today, one may say, has never really died, just divided in two, many times, over the millennia—an immortal entity until the last (the first) is finally stepped on. By contrast, the death of a particular group of cells within a multicellular society may result in the demise of all, regardless of how healthy they were to begin with (as when a person dies of a gunshot wound to the heart or to the brain). This represents the forfeiture of a very important principle: the ability (and purpose) of a single cell to maintain and protect its own life. This commitment to cellular societies is at the core of what we are as multicellular beings, where the individual cell replaces its own survival principles with that of the society. In a multicellular organism, individual cells cannot break their ties to the group and swim away when the going gets tough; this ability has been cashed in.

By becoming multicellular societies, cells exchange one set of freedoms for another: the freedom to negotiate singly and face life's perils alone is exchanged for the freedom to "unionize" and group negotiate, and in so doing, to lose or win as a group.

A second prerequisite for animal evolution was the development of a system for delivering high-energy fuels to hungry cells trapped and packed into immobile arrangements. Essential steps included oxidative metabolism and a digestive system capable of supplying high-level nutrients to very densely packed cell groups via a circulatory system. Thus single cells devoid of an exoskeleton (unlike plants) cannot survive outside of a watery environment having certain nutrients. Eukaryotes cannot survive for long without oxygen. Animals have solved the problem by trapping this all-important fluid environment within, and carrying their internal ocean (blood and extracellular fluid) with them.

A third likely reason why evolution took so long to develop animals is cellular complexity. Think of what must actually be entailed in bringing true cell-to-cell communication into existence. Initially, cells of different genetic lineage develop a biomolecular language, giving rise to a ruled commonality, an all life encompassing bio-politic. In essence, cells had to acquire the ability through trial and error to receive, interpret, and send clear signals among themselves. They did this first, perhaps, as daughter cells of a mutual cell division, held together by the retention of cytoplasmic "bridges" from incomplete separation, or a mucopolysaccharide "glue" on their surfaces (as seen in the primitive cell colony volvox; for reference, see Kirk 1998). Later, they were together as somewhat more distant but genetically close relatives, as heterogeneous cell groups, then as a colony, and finally as a homogeneous group having the same genetic code but each expressing only part of it, and so allowing the cellular specialization mentioned above.

The question arises: what is gained, from an evolutionary perspective, from this new philosophy of order? And the answer is obvious; cell groups have emergent properties that single cells cannot attain. Among these is the ability of individual cells in the group to differentiate, that is, to become specialized for specific tasks (at the expense of their own autonomy) to an extent not possible in a single-cell life form where all requirements for survival must be present in the single element.

Early "Fire"—Single Cells Began to Use Intracellular and Extracellular "Tools"

A great advance in cell-to-cell communication came from the ability that cells evolved to control the concentration of intracellular calcium ion (Kretsinger 1996, 1997; Pietrobon et al. 1990; Williams 1998). Calcium is one of the most reactive elements in the periodic table; it is an extremely difficult ion to tame. At the salinity of the ocean, one finds that calcium is buffered at 10 millimolar or 0.4 grams/liter (that is, the concentration of dissolved calcium ion is 0.4 grams/liter of seawater). Above that concentration, the high reactivity of calcium results in crystal formation (calcium phosphate and carbonate), leading to such things as marble or shells. Thus calcium cannot attain concentrations in water as high as sodium or potassium (in the 100s of millimolar range) without making "rock," and rocks and other crystals are the antithesis of life.

And yet nature has evolved calcium as a requirement for life—and has learned to regulate it with great precision. How did this intensely reactive element weave its way into the fabric of eukaryotic life? It did so as a consequence of its dangerous love affair with another element, phosphorus (Kretsinger 1996, 1997).

Phosphorus is critical to eukaryotic life. Eukaryotic organisms that must support energetically expensive tasks such as muscular contraction and the activity of nerve cells require a means of obtaining the highest levels of usable energy from fuel molecules, and oxygen is essential for this task through the process of oxidative phosphorylation. But in order to keep phosphorus on board for oxidative phosphorylation, eukaryotic life had to learn to fend off the highly reactive calcium. Otherwise, calcium would steal phosphorus from the cell and crystallize, thus stealing life. It is the best of Shakespearean tragedies: the charged event has to be prevented. Eukaryotes dealt with the threat of calcium by developing molecules that recognize and bind calcium, thus preventing it from moving freely within the cell and protecting against potential, dangerous liaisons with phosphorus.

We may come to see that calcium was to the eukaryotic cell what fire was to early humans. Our ancestors needed to control fire, and their relation had to be "neither too close nor too far." The control of fire made us a very powerful animal indeed. Just as we learned to control fire, eukaryotes learned to control calcium. Evolution took advantage of the calmodulin harness on calcium and began to use the reactivity of this element for exceedingly useful purposes.

Once phosphorus was left safely alone to carry out its role in oxidative phosphorylation, oxygen could then be carried efficiently and utilized by eukaryotic cells. With the development of calmodulin, the calcium/calmodulin complex became a serious intracellular tool as a very sophisticated signaling system, and the normally very low concentration of free calcium inside the cell allowed it to be exploited for what we now term "second messenger roles." These roles are of critical importance in conveying information that regulates the triggering of the rapid and localized enzymatic reactions leading to many events such as muscle cell contraction, axon elongation, synaptic transmission, and programmed cell death. This paramount event in eukaryotic evolution provided the biological necessities that allowed for cells to be part of an organized, intercommunicating society.

Neurons Arose within the Space between Sensing and Moving; This Space Mushroomed to Become the Brain

For the next stage in this drama we may revisit the sea squirt, a sessile sea plant rooted to the bottom of the ocean and filter-feeding its life away. When the time has come to reproduce itself, the sea squirt does so by budding, casting off larvae that are, for a brief time, free-swimming tunicates. As I said before, these little fellows are well equipped to negotiate the demands of swimming, as they have on board a primitive "brain" (one or more ganglia), a rudimentary "eye," and an organ for balance (Romer 1969). Once free from the sessile adult, the tadpole-like larva swims off, finds a nook or cranny, parks its head end into it, literally digests most of its own brain, and reverts to the more primitive, sessile adult form of the species. The take-home lesson for us here is that a brain is necessary only for actively moving creatures.

Now consider the evolutionary pressure that would bring about a nervous system. We can look at a primitive, brainless creature such as the Portuguese man-o'-war and see the basic, driving concept already in play (figure 4.2). A man-o'-war is what is known as a "super-organism," which means that it is actually a colony of interdependent, yet genetically unrelated organisms. These organisms are actually themselves cell colonies made up of genetically related cells. Some of these are specialized for buoyancy, some for protection of the colony as a whole, still others for the purposes of reproduction and feeding. But there is cellular communication amongst these elements or individual colonies and so, although

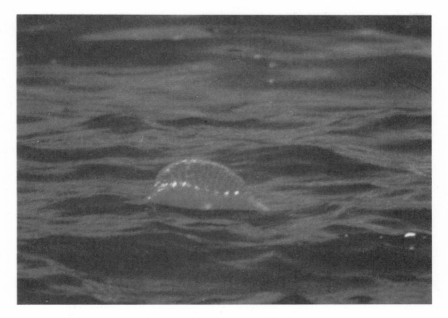

Figure 4.2
Portuguese man-o'-war. Found typically in tropical and subtropical regions of the Pacific and Indian Oceans, and Gulfstream of the Northern Atlantic. Its buoyancy at the surface is due to a gas-filled bladder-like float, 3–12 inches long. Under this float are clusters of polyps from which hang tentacles. The tentacles may be as much as 30 feet long (in some species, 165 feet). The tentacles bear stinging structures that paralyze small fish and other prey. (From websites www.best5.net/animal/Viewlmg/ and www.britannica.com/seo/p/portuguese-man-of-war)

brainless—having no centralized neural networkings—the man-o'-war is capable of considerable coordination.

How can this be? Because the distinct cell colonies comprising the man-o'-war have organized themselves in such a way that "sensory" elements (cells that sense differing forms of energy—mechanical, thermal, etc.) and "motor" elements (cells that generate retraction of the tentacles) are related to one another—even in the absence of a nervous system. Such connectedness of sensory and motor function can be seen every few minutes as the sides of the jellyfish's bright blue float are drawn under the surface of the water to re-moisten the tissues of the gas chamber; the sensory cue here is presumably a degree of tissue "dryness."

If we look at the sensorimotor transformations in a very primitive multicellular organism, say a sponge, we see that the motile cells (cells that generate movement) also respond directly to sensory stimulation with a wave of contraction: touch it, it moves, and in the same way each and every time. The size of the response is basically proportional to the size of the stimulus. We see this form of direct sensorimotor coupling in many land plants as well. Moving up the evolutionary ladder, if we look at the cellular mechanisms of a sea anemone, the sensory and contractile functions that were combined into one type of cell, as in the sponge, have now begun their evolutionary segregation into two distinct elements. One cell, serving the sensory function, responds to stimuli by generating an electrical impulse (or series of impulses, depending on the size of the stimulus); that impulse triggers the motor element or the contractile cell to do its job. The interesting thing to note here is that the sensory cell has become specialized in its function: it is no longer capable of generating movement on its own, but rather has taken on the select role of the reception and transmission of information. In this regard, it is also similar to a motor neuron in that it serves only to drive muscle or motor cell contraction. The next evolutionary step is to insert a motor neuron between the sensory cells and the motor cells. Here, the motor neuron serves to activate muscle fibers, but responds only to the activation of the sensory cell.

The Interneuron

As the evolution of the central nervous system progresses, we see the appearance and juxtaposition of another neuron between the sensory neurons and the motor neurons. These cells are called "interneurons." In a strict sense one may define an interneuron as any nerve cell that does not communicate directly with the world outside the nervous system. Interneurons send and receive signals by means of synaptic contacts to and from other neurons exclusively, and serve to reroute and distribute sensory input to different components of the motor system (the motor neurons and the muscle cells they innervate). If we look at the vertebrate spinal cord, we see interneurons in place, distributing the sensory information they receive to the motor neurons or to other neurons in the central nervous system. The great advantage provided by such often widely branching interneurons is the ability to "steer with multiple reins." The sensory stimuli activating a few sensory cells may activate a small set of interneurons, which may in turn and, through many spinal segments of connectivity, evoke a complex motor response involving a large number of contractile elements. Through this profusely branching forward connectivity, the animal becomes capable of performing well-defined gross movements that involve many muscles along its body.

One should not think of interneurons as a species of neuron that only lives in the spinal cord. Interneurons are found throughout the central nervous system, and there may be many, not just one, juxtaposed between the sensory cell and the motor neuron. If we stick to our definition of an interneuron as any nerve cell that does not communicate directly with the outside world, then the thalamocortical cells (and corticothalamic for that matter) are interneurons as well. In fact, in that sense, the overwhelming majority of neurons comprising our brain are interneurons (figure 4.3). In modern terms, interneurons are defined as neurons that do not project their axons outside the realm (brain region) in which they live, and so they are also called local circuit neurons. Those that contact other brain regions are known as projection neurons. When thought of in this light, it becomes even clearer that for the most part the brain functions as a closed system most of the time. This intricately woven mass of neurons operates as a closed system to perform sensorimotor transformations. Information is fed into this system from the external world, and the results of the operations are put back out into the external world as active, purposeful movement that is necessary for survival. These neurons are the functional space where movement strategies are generated and then implemented; these neurons are where we think.

Nerve Cells and Their Personalities

So what is a neuron then? Neurons or nerve cells constitute a remarkable specialization of the eukaryotic cells that allowed the evolution of natural "computation" by cellular ensembles. Once evolved, they became the central structure in all brains of all animal forms: the carriers of information, the constructors, supporters, and memorizers of an internal

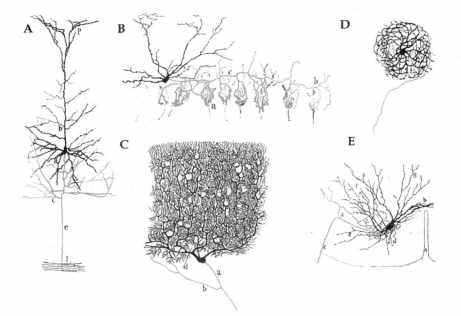

Figure 4.3
Drawings of neurons of the brain and spinal cord. (*A*) Pyramidal cell in the cerebral cortex of a rabbit. (*B*) Basket cell of the cerebellum, with axons that terminate in a basket-like configuration on the cell bodies of many Purkinje cells. (*C*)
Purkinje cell from the human cerebellum. (*C*) Inferior olive cell. (*E*) Fetal cat spinal cord motor neuron with an axon exiting the spinal cord through the ventral
root to terminate on a muscle. (After Ramón y Cajal, 1911.)

world—an internal world composed of neurons that simulates the external reality, stealing from it its principles of operation and injecting back
into the external world the product of cognition.

Neurons came into existence in order to facilitate and orchestrate the
ever-growing complexity of sensorimotor transformations. But how do
they do this? How does a neuron work?

A neuron is essentially a battery, and like a battery, it can generate a
voltage (figure 4.4). This voltage is known as the "membrane potential."
The separation of ionic species (positively and negatively charged atoms
such as sodium and potassium, and also charged large impermeable molecules) inside relative to outside of the neuron that sets up and maintains
the voltage difference. This charge separation occurs because of the

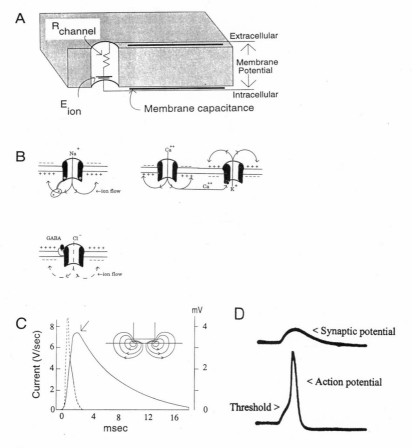

Figure 4.4

Basic electrical properties of the membrane of excitable cells, including neurons and muscle fibers. (*A*) The membrane can be modeled as a battery, with a resistor and capacitor in parallel. Embedded in the membrane are ligand- and voltage-activated ion channels that selectively allow current flow across the membrane. The direction of current flow through a channel when open depends on the potential across the membrane, the charge of the permeable ion, and the concentration gradient of that ion between the inside and outside of the cell. (*B*) Examples of ion channels. The Na^+ and Ca^{2+} channels shown are voltage-activated, while the K^+ and Cl^- channels are ligand-gated (Ca^{2+} and the neurotransmitter GABA, respectively). (*C*) Example of the time course of membrane potential change of an excitatory postsynaptic potential (EPSP, arrow, mV scale at right), which is produced by a short-lasting current (dashed line, scale at left). The rate of fall of the voltage across the membrane depends on the resistive and capacitative properties of the membrane "battery." (*D*) Action potential (bottom trace) triggered by the synaptic potential (upper trace) from "threshold" level. The resting membrane potential for each trace is the level before the onset of the synaptic potential.

existence of large, charged molecules that cannot traverse the cell membrane (are "impermeant"), and the presence of tiny channels in the neuronal membrane, each specific for the passage of only certain ions. Some channels are always open; some only open transiently. There are many factors that determine an individual channel's state at a given moment. This is why one refers to the neuronal membrane as "semi-permeable." Neurons also actively "pump" certain ions in and certain other ions out of the cell against their electrochemical gradients (see below), maintaining the charge separation of inside with respect to outside of this semi-permeable membrane (for general review of ion channels, see Hille 1992).

Given the different ionic environment inside versus outside of the cell, when a channel opens the specific ionic type that is allowed through the channel may flow across. The rate of movement of a charged particle (here through the channel) creates an electrical current and so, when one speaks of a "potassium membrane current," one refers to that electrical current carried by potassium ions as they move through a transiently open "potassium channel" that spans a neuron's membrane. Such a current may be inward or outward, depending on the direction of the "driving force" acting on a given ion. This driving force is set up by an electrochemical gradient.

Opposites attract, and so positively charged ions seek a negative environment, and negatively charged ions seek a positive environment (i.e., are more likely to move toward a positive environment): they move toward electrical neutrality. This, then, is the electrical part of the gradient. Ions also prefer equal concentrations: if the concentration of, say, sodium ions is higher on one side of the membrane, sodium ions will, if given access, cross the membrane and even up the distribution. Let me hasten to say that ions do not "will" their movement; all they can do is move by the simple random walk known as diffusion. The net effect of their random movement is to eliminate concentration differences between the regions. If there are more ions in one region of space, the probability that any ion in the region of higher concentration will move into a region of lower concentration is greater than the probability of the less numerous ions in the lower concentration region moving into regions of greater concentration. This is the chemical part of the gradient. And so, the combined electrical drive and concentration differences inside with respect to outside of the cell determine ionic direction—if it can flow. Whether or not the ion can flow at all brings up the issue of permeability.

Ionic Channels

If an ionic channel across the cell's membrane "opens," it represents a path for given ions to move. This channel is said to be "permeable" to a particular type or types of ion (ionic species differ in their size and charge, and so an open sodium channel will not pass the slightly larger potassium ion); if the channel is closed, it becomes impermeable to that particular ion. The size of a membrane current, then, is determined by the rate of movement of ions through their respective channel. This rate is based on three things: first, that the respective channel be open; second, that the appropriate ion species for the open channel be present (this is called the channel selectivity); and third, that there be a driving force acting on the given ion (it will move down its electrochemical gradient). If there is no driving force acting to move an ion in or out of the cell, there is no net movement of charge and thus no current flows.

And so we can see that membrane voltage is due to a maintained charge separation by a semipermeable membrane that allows passage of only certain ions down their electrochemical gradients via ion-selective channels. There are other ion-moving proteins (enzymes) in this membrane that actively pump certain ions in and certain ions out of the cell (a process differing from the first in that it takes place against an ion's electrochemical gradient, and thus requires work). In the so-called "resting cell"—that is when a neuron is not firing its all-or-none signal, the action potential—this voltage is referred to as the "resting membrane potential." The resting potential is typically on the order of −70 millivolts (mV) with respect to the outside of the cell, which is arbitrarily given as 0 mV. Due to certain electrical events in and about the membrane, a neuron can become depolarized, meaning that its membrane potential changes in a positive direction toward 0 mV, or that its negative potential decreases. A cell can also become hyperpolarized, the membrane polarization increasing to values more negative than −70 mV. There is a particular voltage level known as "threshold," which occurs at values positive to the resting potential, somewhere close to −55 mV. When the membrane becomes depolarized to −55 mV, due to movement of positive charge into the neuron (which adds up over time and membrane area), a set of voltage-dependent channels opens for a very short time (activated only at particular membrane voltages). These newly opened channels cause more positive charge to flow in (a chain reaction), which results in the generation of an action potential: a short-lasting (one-thousandth of a second) single depolarizing wave that grows in amplitude very fast until it can grow no more, as the driving force for ion movement is exhausted. The action potential is about 100 mV in amplitude (-70 mV to a positive potential around $+30$ mV with respect to the outside) that travels down the axon in a self-regenerating fashion.

The Action Potential

The action potential is termed "all-or-none" because like any expulsion it either occurs or fails. This character is due to its chain reaction nature, which forces it to be as large as possible given the driving force. Once activated, it travels down the axon without changing in size, and once initiated, it is difficult to stop. This action potential, or "spike," is a soliton, an electric wave that travels (as a wave in a whip) from the cell body at a site known as the "axon hillock" down the axon to the "axon terminals." These terminals each contact other neurons, forming "synapses." Although nerve terminals may form synapses with any region of the target neuron, the most common point of contact is with the target cell's dendrites. Dendrites are branching projections that also serve as the antennae that receive impulses from other neurons. The number of individual synapses on a given dendritic "tree" can easily be in the tens of thousands. The dendrites conduct these incoming synaptic currents, which are either positive or negative, down the dendritic "branches," to its "trunk" and into the cell body. There, these potentials, positive and negative, are summed over time across the membrane, and if positive outweighs negative, enough to depolarize the cell to -55 mV, this cell will fire its action potential (figure 4.4D).

One should not get the impression that this all-or-none action potential stays that way from neuron to neuron; this is not the case. When the action potential reaches the axon terminals of the presynaptic neuron, this depolarization causes (again, through voltage-dependent mechanisms) the release of neurotransmitters. As mentioned previously, these special molecules are intercellular messengers that diffuse across the space between the two cells, the "synaptic cleft" (figure 4.5) (neurons are not

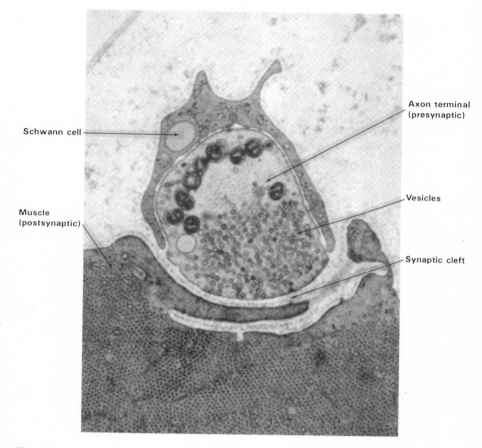

Schwann cell

Axon terminal
(presynaptic)

Muscle
(postsynaptic)

Vesicles

Synaptic cleft

Figure 4.5
Electron micrograph showing a motor neuron axon terminal forming a neuromuscular junction on a muscle fiber. The axon terminal contains synaptic vesicles, small packets filled with neurotransmitter molecules, that release their contents into the space between the presynaptic (axonal) and postsynaptic (muscle) elements during synaptic transmission. The neurotransmitter molecules diffuse across the interstitial space, or synaptic cleft, and bind to receptors on the muscle membrane, triggering the opening of ion channels that depolarize the membrane, generating a synaptic potential. If the synaptic potential results in a large enough depolarization, an action potential is triggered that initiates the cascade of events leading to muscle contraction. The hexagonally arranged dots seen in the muscle are cross-sectional views of myofibrils, which contain the contractile machinery of the muscle fiber. (Kindly provided by Dr. T. Reese.)

actually physically connected; the fluid-filled space between them is approximately 20 nanometers, or 20×10^{-9} meters) and bind to specific receptors on the membrane of the receiving or postsynaptic neuron. When activated in this fashion, these receptors cause changes in the dynamics of associated ion channels in the membrane of the postsynaptic cell, usually at a dendrite. These changes alter the flow of ions through the dendritic membrane, thereby generating small currents that cause small voltage shifts—called "synaptic potentials"—in the local area of the membrane.

Synaptic Potentials

Synaptic potentials are also called graded potentials. Unlike the action potential, synaptic potentials vary in size from fractions of a millivolt to tens of millivolts. They are produced by the release of small amounts of transmitter from vesicles (quanta), each of which is known as a miniature potential (figure 4.6, upper left). The sum of many of these small membrane polarizations make up the synaptic potentials that are subject to decay along the postsynaptic membrane, in that they are not observed a short distance away from the synaptic junction (figure 4.6, upper right). They are local events that can trigger chain reaction events while lacking such properties themselves.

Indeed, while synaptic potentials are individually small, they will sum together to make larger potentials. If there are enough of these events within a short time period to outweigh the decay processes as they are conducted toward the cell body (such processes are called the cable properties of the membrane), they may add to depolarize the cell to −55 mV, and off goes an action potential in the receiving cell (figure 4.6A).

The transfer of signals from one neuron to another is first electrical, in the action potential, then chemical, in synaptic transmission, and then electrical again with the generation of the next action potential. This is why neuronal communication is called "electrochemical coupling" or "electrochemical signaling."

Electrotonic Coupling

We spoke of electrotonic coupling in chapter 2; it was shown that this form of neuronal communication allows the inferior olivary nucleus to oscillate in phase as a singular ensemble of neurons. As opposed to the

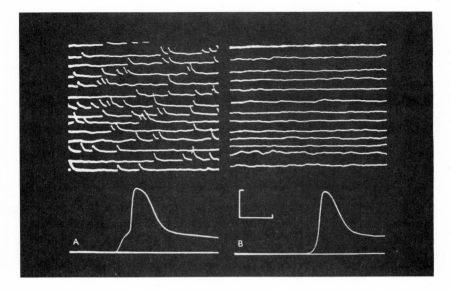

Figure 4.6

Intracellular recordings made inside a muscle fiber near to (left) and remote from (right) a neuromuscular junction (nmj). (*Top*) Recording of spontaneous synaptic potentials (miniature excitatory postsynaptic potentials, MEPPs) representing the release of neurotransmitter from a single synaptic vesicle released from the nerve terminal. At right, no synaptic potentials are recorded because of the location of the electrode remote to the synaptic site. The decrementing synaptic potentials can only be recorded near to the synaptic site. (*Bottom*) Recording of synaptic potential and action potential it triggers near to (left) and remote from (right) the synaptic site. At right, the synaptic potential is not seen due to the location of the recording electrode far from the site of origin of the decrementing signal. The action potential is recorded because it is regeneratively propagated down the membrane to the remote location of the recording electrode. See text for more details. (From Fatt and Katz, 1952.)

chemical synapse where the diffusional space between neurons, the synaptic cleft, is on the order of 20 nanometers, neurons forming electrotonic connections come into much closer apposition and generate bridges between them. This electrically conductive bridge is called a gap junction (Bennett 1997, 2000). At such junctions between two (or more) neurons there are gap junction channels. If one injects fluorescent dye into one of these connected neurons, the flow of dye is unimpeded through these channels and thus between cells. These gap junction channels allow conduction of ions (electric current) directly between the cells, thus making them electrically coupled. There are no neurotransmitters in electrotonic flow and so there is very little, if any, delay in the voltage shifts imparted by the flow of electricity from one cell to another. The process of electrochemical signaling has associated with it a small delay due to the many steps involved in the release of transmitter, diffusion time across the cleft, subsequent transmitter binding, and then activation of the associated ion channels to allow current flow in and out of the local area of the membrane. This all takes anywhere from 1 to 5 milliseconds. With electrotonic connectivity, however, the ionic flow is through channels that are already open (although they can close), and current flows between cells directly as the interior of the cells are interconnected. Consequently, when one neuron fires an action potential, any cell electrotonically coupled to it is compelled to receive part of the signal, virtually simultaneously, and if the signal is large enough, it will itself fire action potentials in the coupled cells.

Is such electrical flow bidirectional? It turns out that many gap junctions regulate current flow in an even, bidirectional manner (Bennett 2000). Bidirectionality is seen in the electrical connections of the inferior olive (IO) cells, which allows such cells to function, electrically, almost as one big cell (for review, see Welsh and Llinás 1997). But not all gap junctions operate in such a bidirectional fashion. Some gap junctions allow ionically carried current flow in only one direction and thus send their signal simultaneously to the next neuron but do not receive signals back from that cell (see Furshpan and Potter 1959).

And so, because of this direct flow of current from cell to cell by means of electrotonic coupling, the result is rapid and synchronous firing of interconnected cells. This is how "ensemble" signaling occurs. These types of signaling allow groups of neurons to convey to widely scattered and perhaps distantly located neurons a concise and synchronous signal pattern. The simultaneity produced by electrical coupling gives this signal the "roar of the masses" as many cells fire together, rather than the "voice in the wilderness" of a single cell. It is a choir as opposed to a solo performance. This issue of temporal binding relates also to the seamlessness we sense in consciousness.

Electrotonic coupling plays a significant role in developmental processes as well. We saw in chapter 3 the advantage of simultaneous signaling in order to internalize motricity from myogenically rhythmic muscles to the function of the oscillatory resonance of the brain itself. Such coupling during development also takes advantage of the fact that the diameters of the gap junction channels are comparatively large (Bennett 2000). In addition to ions, gap junctions allow flow of relatively large molecules that play important, internal regulatory roles in development and cell function, and which might have a harder time getting into the cells otherwise, given their size. The gap junction channels are roughly 1.5 nm in diameter, allowing small peptides and also critical molecules such as cyclic adenosine monophosphate (cAMP) to pass from cell to cell (see Simpson et al. 1977; Pitts and Sims 1977; Kam et al. 1998; Bevans et al. 1998). Such larger molecules cannot pass into cells by way of the ion channels in the cell's membrane, as these channels are simply much too small. One may look at this as a form of regulatory simultaneity between developing neurons.

And so, the basic functional unity for the neuron is electrical, with electrotonic interactions and action potentials serving as the temporal binding element giving the neuron its integrative backbone. Chemical and electrical synaptic transmission are, on the other hand, the basic coinage that binds the different cellular elements into single multicellular functional states.

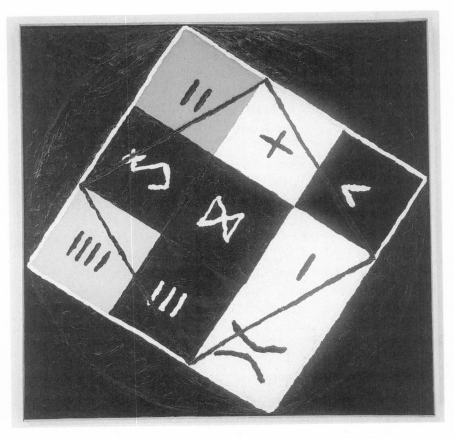

Alfred Jensen, *Square Beginning—Cyclic Ending, Per I–V,* 1960. Oil on canvas, 50 × 250 in., overall; five panels, 50 × 50 in each; panel 4. Courtesy of PaceWildenstein. Photograph by Ellen Page Wilson.

5

Lessons from the
Evolution of the Eye

The Invention of Sensory Organs

What is the evolutionary drive to form an animal? How is such a spectacular and complex cellular-based architecture generated? And what can
one say of organs and their vast diversity of form and function within an
animal? We think of our organs from a perspective of physiological division of labor, as specialized components of our bodies whose functional
roles are unique, often singularly so. In most cases they are vital to the organism as a whole, in the short run of a given lifetime and in the long run
for the perpetuation of the species. The heart, the eyes, the liver—they are
modules, individual local devices. In many ways, like the brain, a given
organ may be considered a specialized, closed society within an animal.
Among these many similarities, however, there is an exceptional difference. The brain is basically closed in its nature and operation. It completely escapes direct examination by any of our senses. We cannot see it,
we cannot hear it, we do not feel it beating, it does not heave up and
down, it can feel no pain if we strike it. And more, it seems capable of being remote from its corporeal anchor—as when we empathize with the
pain of others or observe with admiration the universe around us.

This closed organic system we call the brain has the further advantage of not being limited by the properties of the senses. Consider that the waking state is a dreamlike state (in the same sense that dreaming is a wakelike state) guided and shaped by the senses, whereas regular dreaming does not involve the senses at all. Although the brain may use the senses to take in the richness of the world, it is not limited by those senses; it is capable of doing what it does without any sensory input whatsoever. The nature of the brain and what it does makes the nervous system a very different type of entity from the rest of the universe. It is, as stated repeatedly, a reality emulator. Suggesting that the system is closed, and so very different, means that it must be another way of expressing "everything." In other words, *brain activity is a metaphor for everything else.* Comforting or disturbing, the fact is that we are basically dreaming machines that construct virtual models of the real world. It is probably as much as we can do with only one and a half pounds of mass and a "dim" power consumption of 14 watts (Erecinska and Silver 1994).

Perhaps more puzzling still is that this unique and specific functional architecture, this closed cellular system, forms without knowing a priori what it or its function is to be! How can *this* be? It turns out that this is one of the curiosities of the evolutionary process that the brain has in common with all organs. They have all developed into their complex and unique structures, their specific and capable functions, without any a priori final plan. "But wait, what about genetics and the developmental plan preprogrammed into our DNA?" you ask. Well, of course genetics are involved, but only as an accumulated result of each generation's storytelling of the great epic, with no overarching plot and certainly no end. There are plenty of characters, a bang of a beginning, but then only a tumbling, churning, never-ending middle. Curious indeed.

How can one understand the process by which the nervous system, the mind, came to us if its ancestry started out in evolution without a compass or a map? Well, all other organs (as the animals they inhabit) developed in the same way, by trial and error, and in a process that has no end.

In order to develop the nervous system nature had to learn from the properties of the external universe and it had to incorporate them in beneficial ways. In chapter 3, the deeply important issue of embedding was discussed. Now it is time to ask what the first step is in this process. How do we take in fractionalized properties of the external world and put them in the context of a single whole? Evolution had to "invent" sensory organs, specialized relay mechanisms between the universals of the external world and the inherently closed system that is the brain. It is perhaps easier to understand that this "taking in" of external properties is precisely what nature has had life do over all of evolution, when we understand the sensory relay or transformation process at the momentary level. Momentary level is, for example, how one may take in patterns of light, right now as you read; these patterns make up the words on this page, which come out somehow as a voice in your head. Rolling through the millennia, the system embeds, "remembers," and what is the result? Primitive photoreceptors functioning to detect light have evolved into the wondrously complex organs that are our eyes. The primitive statocyst, that at one stage was (and still is) the rudimentary balancing mechanism for the sea squirt, has evolved into the enormously important and intricately networked subsystem of the brain we call the vestibular system. Sensory systems have evolved as exceedingly sophisticated tools for the brain, honed over the eons to ever increase and perfect the proficiency of predictive movement and thus survival.

Our descriptions imply a slant toward sensory organs. This is the case, but it needn't be so. The learning from the embedding of the universal properties of the external world drove the formation of all organs, as well as feet and hands, tails and feathers. But with sensory organs, this process is easier to understand because sensory organs are direct conduits from the external world to the internal world of the brain, and the brain is the attracting focus of this book. The liver, for example, evolved under these same principles of evolutionary pressure but in ways somewhat less direct. The liver evolved to help rid our systems of toxins that we unwittingly (or some times wittingly, as with the fondness for wine) take in. But toxicity is mainly relative across species; it is not a *universal*. What makes us deathly ill is a happy snack for a rat or a beetle's daily routine. When I speak of universal properties, or simply universals, I am referring to those properties arising from the external world that are invariant across all of life. Light waves, for example, have a universal property, as does temperature or the force of gravity. These are among the very first, powerful, unchanging phenomena that life had to confront and by which life has been shaped. But can all this be understood? Well, let us think of one function—seeing—and one set of organs—the eyes.

Why Eyes?

As mentioned above, I am slanting toward sensory organs, and in this chapter eyes are my central example, because of the variety of forms that have evolved for the transduction (conversion) of light into useful specification of internal brain states. Basically, in all cases and for all the senses, the brain only accepts those specific properties of the external world that stimulate sense organs (we do not sense radio or TV electromagnetic waves directly) and these inputs are conveyed only as neuronal electrical activity.

So to Begin, What Is Vision?

What does it mean to "see"? Why is the visual apparatus the way it is and what can it teach us about the brain—the *mind*? (For an excellent review of vision consult Zeki 1993.)

The eye (figure 5.1A), and in particular the retina (the light-sensitive part), is a true extension of the central nervous system (figure 5.1B). The neurons in the retina form an extraordinarily compact and beautiful circuit that sends the electrical messages that the brain interprets as light. In chapter 4, we came to understand that it is not just the ensemble properties of neuronal circuits that give rise to a particular circuit's unique and specific behavior and function; it is the architecture of the ensemble that gives the circuit its macroscopic properties (as in the case of the heart) and through such architectures both context and intentionality. These architectures, or modules, are generally formed by neuronal elements of different types and of different intrinsic electrical properties. Some are excitatory and some inhibitory. In the case of the eye, the retina provides an excellent example of this strategy. So with our eyes and our mind's eye, let's take a look into the evolution of the eye, *our eye,* and some other fascinating eyes as well.

It all began with organisms taking advantage of the energy from the sun. Solar energy is absolutely essential for life. We are on earth courtesy

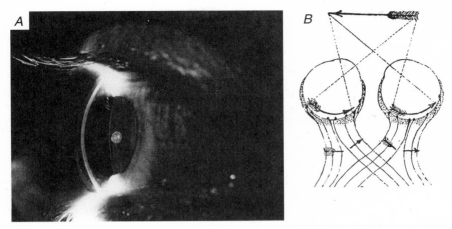

Figure 5.1
(*A*) Photograph of the human eye in profile. Light enters the eye through the transparent cornea, where much of the bending of light takes place. The white dot on the pupil is a reflection of light. (From Hubel, 1988, p. 35.) (*B*) Simplified diagram of neuronal organization of the retina. (From Cajal, 1911, figure 571.)

of the vegetable kingdom, the first sun-worshiping group. Plants and trees and green algae took a direct road by evolving to convert light/solar energy into *food*—hence the name of this process, *photosynthesis*. Photosynthesis provides the means for the plant to form carbohydrates, proteins, and fats. Thus, plants and trees and green algae make their own food, a very clever solution. Animals, on the other hand, are more devious. They convert light energy into *neuronal signaling,* the patterns of activity that let them "see," and then they eat the plants (and each other).

Why don't plants and green algae "see"? As pointed out before, it stems from the fact that they don't move, or in the case of the algae, not at a rate that could get them into any trouble—or out of it, for that matter. They make their own food and they "mate" by scattering their seeds, or by cross-pollination, or by dividing. They have an effective survival strategy without being able to move actively. As far as plants are concerned, predators may be warded off by thorns and chemical repellents. Given the predators that plants and trees have to contend with, an ability to move actively would probably not help much. Parasites go with you, locusts and woodpeckers both fly, and it is doubtful that a tree, given the miraculous ability to fly or move at all, would be able to outrun either.

So trees do not run or fly and they cannot beat off enemies with their branches. The closest that trees come to moving would be what is called phototropism, the tendency for such photophilic life forms to bend toward light, or drift, as the case may be for the algae. But this is more accurately thought of in terms of the Jamesian reflexology we discussed in chapter 2, rather than any form of self-referential movement. Trees do not move actively, and that is why they neither need, nor have, a brain: their survival does not depend on prediction.

As for actively moving creatures, "teleception," or remote sensing such as seeing, hearing, or smelling, extends a creature's predictive capacity in negotiating the external world. It is nice to be able to see that a threat is coming, as opposed to having to feel it through one's outer being first, or perhaps to have to taste it, in order to register belatedly its arrival. Indeed, we sense these latter modes of sensory transduction, information through feeling and tasting, as being, in the context of an oncoming predator, too close. For us, too close in these cases usually means too late. And so teleception, remote sensing, arose to buy more time for prediction and the predictive properties of the brain to be useful.

The earliest aspects of prediction that gave rise to the magnificent organs we know as eyes started with the need of very early creatures to sense light. In the ocean, the need was to predict which way was up to the surface and which down to the depths. In terrestrial forms, the need was for safety, as one knows from seeing a speeding cockroach disappear into the woodwork as one turns on the light at night when looking for a snack. Hiding in the dark usually works out better than hiding in the sun. Originally these basic but clear needs had nothing to do with seeing an image, or even of forming one; they were simply the need to sense whether or not there was light. At this stage, the ability to sense the *direction* of a light source, although incredibly helpful, required an organ yet to evolve. To understand this transition of organ capability—the detection of light versus the detection of the direction of a light source—we have to look into the phototransduction process itself.

Light is made up of events called photons. The argument continues as to whether photons are particles that act like waves or waves that act like particles or neither. From a physiological perspective, we consider them to be energy packets (quanta) that activate a receptor, but the *wavelength* of these electromagnetic quanta emitted by the sun is critical as well; differing wavelengths of photons translate to us as different *colors*.

These wavelike particles travel in straight lines at close to 300,000 kilometers/second. Because photons interact with each other and reinforce or cancel one another (Richard Feynman's "Sum Over Histories" in Feynman and Hibbs, 1965), even if light reflects off something, it nevertheless continues to travel straight. Light can also be refracted, which means that as it passes from one medium to another (say from air to water or glass), its angle of trajectory can be changed as it passes through. After the light is set on this new path, it remains straight as long as the medium does not change or as long as the space in which it travels is not warped by a big gravitational field. The angular degree to which a medium bends the trajectory of light is known as its "refractive index." The higher the degree of bending, the higher the index.

Thus light can bounce off things, as in reflection, and it can pass through things, as in refraction, and so light can inform us of the optical properties of the universe around us. Light can be caught or absorbed. The fact that light travels in a straight line is particularly important, as it means that it is easy to work with light and easy to know its source. The facts that light follows a straight trajectory and is abundant, were essential in the evolution of vision, enabling photons striking the eye to function as accurate and faithful messengers communicating to us the remote landscape of the external world.

Photons are "caught" by pigmented matter. Or rather, matter is pigmented (colored) because it absorbs particular photons. Pigments are what give color to things, and it works as follows. As mentioned before, light photons come in different wavelengths. A traveling light beam has a sinusoidal character, like waves in water, a certain distance from peak to peak (or trough to trough) known as wavelength. For the range of colors we can see, called the visible spectrum, these wavelengths are in the hundreds of nanometers (nms) or 10^{-9} meters. For instance, what we see as blue is light in the 420-nm wavelength range; red is in the longer 550-nm wavelength range.

One may also refer to the frequency of light. Frequency is inversely related to wavelength: the longer the wavelength, the lower the frequency. Frequency is a measure of the number of individual wave cycles in a second. If the space between peaks is greater, that is, the wavelength is longer, then it stands to reason that fewer wave cycles will pass by some given point in a second, and thus the frequency will be lower. Frequency is not the same as speed. The speed of light, for the purposes at hand, does not change. It is a constant.

Natural sunlight is a mixture of all the light frequencies of the entire color spectrum. And so, is it my colleague's blue book in front of me that is absorbing blue light, or is it my eye? It is the eye that is catching the blue light. If it were the book that absorbed the blue light, how would the blueness information reach my brain? The pigment in the dictionary cover has absorbed, stopped, or caught the color frequencies *other* than blue. Blue has been reflected off, and in a straight line; the photons of this frequency have made it to my eye. However, keep in mind that blueness does not exist in the external world. Blueness is a brain interpretation given to a particular wavelength (420 nm) range.

It is my eye that is absorbing—stopping—these photons of light whose frequency says "blue." How is this done? The photons were absorbed by neurons called photoreceptors. In these photoreceptors are found a class of very old proteins called opsins, a component of the visual pigment. These opsins interact closely with a second molecule called a chromophore (the actual photon catcher), triggering the activation of the receptor cell when light strikes. In the case of my colleague's book, as the higher proportion of blue photons were reflected toward me, a greater proportion of blue photon-catching photoreceptors were activated.

Now let's go back to our primitive creature who is just trying to sense light photons, a patch of photosensitive skin, photoreceptors, reflection, and refraction

Photon Sensing and the Direction of Light

The photoreceptor neuron determines light intensity by "counting" the number of photons it catches. Each time a photon is caught, the membrane potential of the photoreceptor changes slightly, so light is measured in incremental membrane potential steps. In fact, we humans can detect at the single photon level (Hubel 1988). The pattern of electrical activity given by a group of photoreceptors counting light photons gives the magnitude of the light received. The changes in the patterns of photoreceptor counting can give a measure of the fluctuation of the light source (shadow, predator). And so we have a primitive creature with a patch of photosensitive skin or "eye spot."

The ability to sense day or night, and perhaps that light meant warmth, was certainly helpful to survival. But can one improve on this? How does one do a better job of catching light? Well, the photosensitive patch of skin, which is actually composed of ciliated ectodermal cells containing some 100 photoreceptors (Land and Fernald 1992), cannot generate an image of what is out there. As this photoreceptor "patch" begins to enlarge in area, however, it tends naturally to form a cup shape or pit. Thus if light comes directly from the front, the back of the cup is activated. Light coming from any other angle will tend to activate the cup asymmetrically, giving rise to a very crude directionality allowing, at most, up and down differentiation, and maybe left and right as well. Many of these pitlike eyes actually only respond to rapid changes in light (moving shadows).

Then a wondrous event occurred in evolution. This cupped patch of skin, containing 100 photoreceptors or so, enlarged further and reduced its aperture (diameter of the opening at the front), closing over to form a cystlike structure. This gave rise to what is known as the "cup eye." The cup eventually became closed completely except for a small hole, and this gave rise to the "pinhole eye," where the pinhole serves as a lens. An inverted real image of the world was projected on to the photoreceptive surface. A better image was achieved when lenses in the form of transparent epithelia finally evolved (Ali 1984) (figure 5.2).

Some Eyes Are Weird

Now we enter the truth-is-stranger-than-fiction realm. My friends Enrico Nasi and Maria del Pilar Gomez, who work during the summers at the Woods Hole Marine Biological Laboratory, are experts on photoreception and study the eyes of scallops. These delicious mollusks have, at the point of contact of their two shells, a large number of beautifully rounded blue eyes that peer in all directions and are, as I learned from Enrico and Maria, quite strange. Unlike our eyes, which have a retina

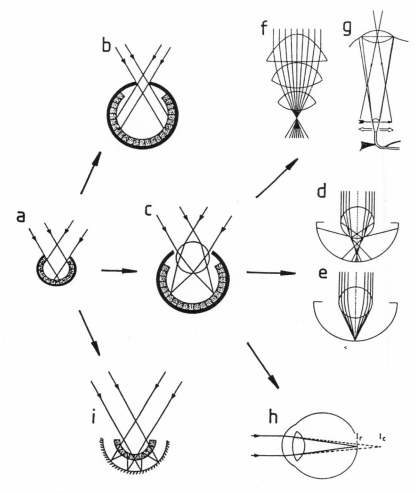

Figure 5.2
Evolution of the single-chambered eye. Arrows indicate structural developments rather than specific evolutionary sequences. (*a*) Pit eye. (*b*) Pinhole eye, found in Nautilus. (*c*) Eye with lens. (*d*) Homogeneous lens. (*e*) Inhomogeneous, "Matthiesen" lens. (*f*) Multiple lens eye of male Pontella. (*g*) Two-lens eye of *Copilia* (see figure 5.4). Solid arrow shows image position. Open arrow, the movement of the scanning second lens. (*h*) Human eye with cornea and lens. Ic, image formed by cornea alone; Ir, final image on retina. (*i*) Mirror eye of the scallop *Pecten*. (From Land and Fernald, 1992, figure 1, p. 6).

against the back end of the eye cup, scallops have two back-to-back retinas that hang in an up-down direction like a projection screen near the center of the eye. This screen divides the eye cup into a front and a back half. These retinas, like two opposing drum skins, are organized so that the front one measures light intensity as the light enters the eye. The light passes through this retina and hits the back of the eye, which is a mirrored surface! Upon hitting the mirror, as in a Newtonian telescope, the light is focused back on to the second retina located at the back of the first one. This second retina receives the light image made by the back mirror. Both retinas send their messages out through an optic nerve that radiates from the eye cup at the equator (if we consider that the north and south poles are respectively the front and back of the eye) (figure 5.3).

They Get Weirder

In some other marine invertebrates such as the ostracod crustacean *Gigantocypris,* the eye consists not of a lens, but a parabolic mirror (figure 5.4). The mirror collects light and focuses it on a match head-like retina (a bit like the front light of a car, if one exchanges the light bulb for a bulb-shaped retina) (Land 1980). And, weirder still, in heteropod sea snails and in jumping spiders, among others, the retina is a strip that is only a few receptors across and several hundred receptors long; the eye scans by tilting the retina through a 90-degree arc (Land and Fernald 1992). But the real weirdo in the eye world is that of *Copilia,* a marine invertebrate found in the Mediterranean near Naples (figure 5.5). This creature has a transparent head-bound immobile lens (like an airplane window). Inside the head there is a second lens and a small group of photoreceptors that scan the horizon five times a second, not unlike the sweep of a television set.

What does all this say? It says that a surface that originally only absorbed light can evolve through a set of intermediate steps that do not yet make images, into one that can support image making! This bit of skin has become a highly specialized module of function: it has become an organ, the eye.

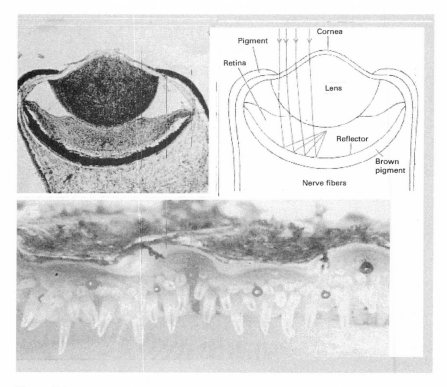

Figure 5.3

The scallop eye. (*Top*) A cross section through this eye shows that, unlike the lens eyes of vertebrates, which have a clear zone between the lens and the retina across which light rays are focused, the lens of the scallop eye is in contact with a crescent-shaped retina. Behind the retina is the extremely thin mirror (not discernible at this magnification) and then a thick layer of dark pigment. At right, a diagram shows the path of light entering this eye. The light, only weakly refracted by the lens, passes through the retina to the hemispherical reflector, which focuses the light back to the distal photoreceptor cells in the upper layer of the retina. Because the light passes through the retina once before it is detected, the contrast acuity of the scallop eye is poor. (*Bottom*) The eyes of the scallop *Pecten* are seen in this photograph as small globules (highlighted by circles) along the mollusk's mantle, which is exposed through the gaping opening of the two valves, or shells. Within each eye, about a millimeter in diameter, is a shiny hemispherical mirror. The eyes detect the movement of a shadow or a dark edge across the animal's field of view, allowing the scallop to discern the approach of a predator. These low-contrast-acuity eyes may also play a role in phototaxis: movement toward areas of darkness or light. (From Land 1978, pp. 127, 130.)

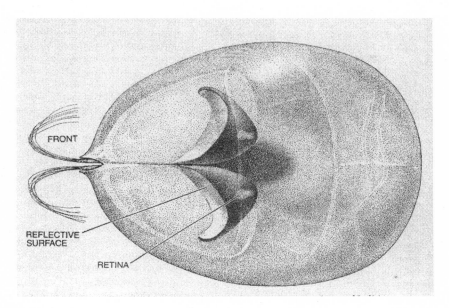

Figure 5.4
Another mirror eye. The deep-sea crustacean *Gigantocypris* has large reflecting eyes that enable it to concentrate the extremely faint light available at a depth of 1,000 meters in the ocean (primarily from the light organs of luminescent crustaceans and fishes). About a centimeter long, this scallop's head makes up about half of its body. The two reflecting eyes are covered by transparent windows in the orange carapace that completely encloses the animal. Sir Alister Hardy of the University of Oxford likened its eyes to the "headlamps of a large car." Hardy was the first to speculate that the mirrors serve to focus light. (From Land, 1978, p. 131)

From Cells Come Systems

And so, from the complexity inherent to cells, the complexity of systems arises. It has done so without knowing *a priori* what it is going to become. These are emergent properties; the systems are not all or none, but evolve. Yet intuitively, it would seem that *something*, some attractor, some process, must lead the eye to become what it is, given its unbelievable complexity. But that is exactly what the process is *not*. There is no intention to become an eye. With the eye, almost every possible solution has been implemented in the wake of its emergence. The

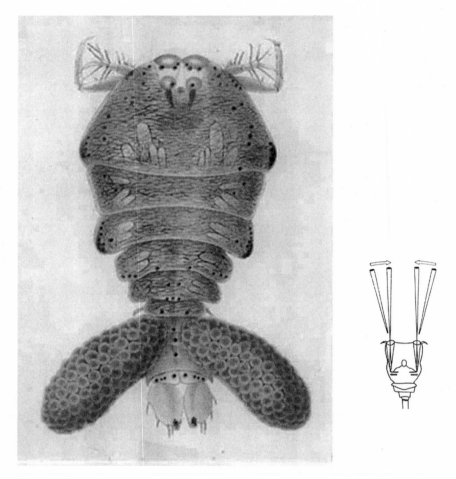

Figure 5.5
(Left) copepod *Copilia* (*Right*) Diagram of the eyes. Retinae subtend only 3″ of arc, and scan through a total of 14″ of arc. (From website nmnhwww.si.edu/iz/copepod/_borders/).

system did not know to do a flat retina or a Galilean lens; it simply tried everything that was feasible structurally, and for which there was some functional advantage at the time. What do all the solutions have in common? They share exploitation of the properties of light, namely that it goes straight and generates an image through reflection or refraction. Once we understand that, we can probably understand every conceivable peripheral visual system, whether here or on another planet.

How is it that we know that evolution has indeed tried almost everything in terms of making images with light? Well, in truth we do not, but it is likely simply because the photoreceptor has been around for such a long time. Or perhaps evolution has not yet tried *everything*, but let's look at it this way. Nature does not design, yet spectacular things happen. Let me give you another example.

Ask yourself, how much does a bag of marbles cost? A few dollars? But people need jobs to make a living, so the actual cost of producing the bag full of marbles must probably be a few pennies. How do you make a marble so perfect, so totally seamless and absolutely spherical, at such a tiny price? And remember, marbles have beautiful patterns in them as well. So how do you do it?

Well, probably for most people, the idea of the shot tower comes to mind. With a shot tower, molten lead is sprayed out and falls into a cooling liquid. As the lead falls, it congeals into more or less spherical bits. Any liquid if tossed from a sufficient height will congeal into spheres. But with marbles, this would be a very expensive approach to their production and you would not be able to incorporate, in any controllable way, the patterns you want the marbles to have. Furthermore, the marbles would not be perfectly round. Instead, the solution is to melt glass, shape it into a rod while it is still soft, put in your patterns, and cut into short cylinders. Then you tumble them together in a tumbling drum with abrasives. After a period of tumbling time, the marbles come out perfectly round, or, at least they approach perfect roundness.

This is precisely what happens in biology, over evolution: if you let something tumble long enough, it comes out almost perfect. Such is the power of random collisions and patience, and that constitutes the sum total of nature's intelligence. All the rough edges, the flaws, the things that don't work are systematically dispatched by natural selection. What remains and carries on into the next generation and the next after that and so on are the advantageous aspects, what *does work, what makes survival easier. And survival is the fuel of natural selection.*

Against this simple view is the fact that in biology developing perfection may never be attained, even with a lot of tumbling.

What does "perfect" mean in biology? It means getting a job done—a particular, *specialized* job like seeing—as efficiently as possible with the lowest possible cost or effort. It means making modules, local apparatuses that give a creature an advantage in negotiating the world, such as an eye that sees or a vestibular system that gives an organism a sense of balance. And it also means that the cost to build such an apparatus over time is as low as possible.

If, for some reason nature found that in order to make an animal's eyes big enough to see in the dark they would hinder its mobility, one would then say that the cost is too high. And nature knows this, which is why you don't see really huge eyes out there. Although I maintain a healthy respect for evolution, I have come to believe that it can be explained basically as a product of the Universal Law of Laziness. This law preaches convenience and usefulness: the path of least resistance. Light is free (daylight, I mean). It doesn't cost a thing to use it. And what happens? If you tumble the evolutionary drive that takes advantage of the fact that light energy is free and easy to catch, you get plants that make their own food, or you get a patch of skin that becomes an eye and can make images of the external world. All of this comes from taking the low road. Take what works and discard what doesn't, and above all avoid risks.

But this actually leads us to a deeper issue. We have an eye that has evolved to make images of the external world from bouncing photons. But what *is* an image? An image is a *simplification of reality.* Our brain is making a simplification of reality. It is making a *simplification* of the external world, but a very useful one. An image is a simplified representation of the external world *written in a strange form.* Any sensory transduction is a simplified representation of a universal arising from the external world. The brain is quite Kantian in the essence of its operation. It makes representations of aspects of the external world, fractionalized aspects, by making a useful geometry, a geometry with internal meaning that has nothing to do with the "geometry" of the external world that gave rise to it. This is the vector/vector transformational capability of the brain that is independent of the coordinate systems utilized to measure it.

Consider colors, which are just the particular way we transduce energy at a particular frequency. A snake sees infrared, which is actually heat. It is very clear that the images in our head are only a representation of the world.

Eyes are neurons that embed geometries of bouncing light, and the brain is a set of coordinate systems that measure or recognize abstract geometries that do not exist in the external world. The smell of the forest is an internal abstraction that does not exist as an external geometry.

Here is a further thought to consider: language is an eye, but an abstract one, an internal abstraction.

Just as a patch of photosensitive skin became an eye, language as we know it followed the same journey. Both are specialized apparatuses for the geometrical internalization of external, fractionalized properties. Thus we have the following streams: patch/wrinkle/cup/pinhole/eye; the generation of protonetworks to the mature functional system, analogous to protolanguage, developing to language (perhaps it still is protolanguage!)

I say that I am a closed system but not a solipsist. I can't be, because of the way I was built by evolution by internalizing the properties of the outside world.

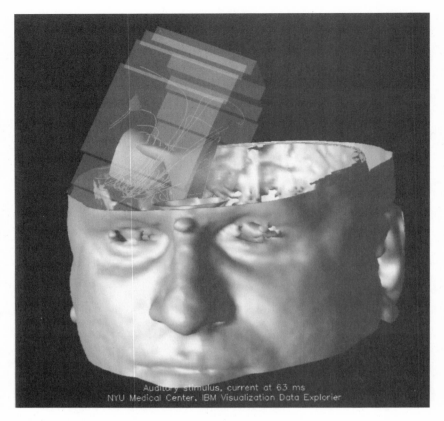

3D imaging scan representing an auditory stimulus (current at 63 ms). Courtesy of NYU Medical Center/Visualization Data Explorer.

6

The I of the Vortex

Consciousness and the Nature of Subjectivity

Having touched briefly on the cell biological rules that evolution has employed to internalize fractured components of the external world (chapters 1–3), we come now to the question of synthesis: how do all these differing components come together into a singular, global, internal construct? Because these neurons of varying "personalities" are by definition relatively specialized (chapter 4), no particular cell's activity can represent more than a small component of such reality. In chapter 5 we saw that photoreceptors are cells specialized for capturing photons and transducing (converting) this electromagnetic energy into electrical activity. Similarly, in our skin we have what are known as mechanoreceptors, specialized cells that transduce mechanical energy into a pattern of neuronal activity (figure 6.1). That you can feel this book in your hands is mediated in part by an array of different mechanoreceptors that tell of pressure, pressure changes, and pressure differences on/to the skin. Working in parallel with these are the joint receptors and muscle sensors known as "muscle spindles" that give you a sense of limb position in space. In short, you don't need to be able to see your hands holding this book to know that you are doing so.

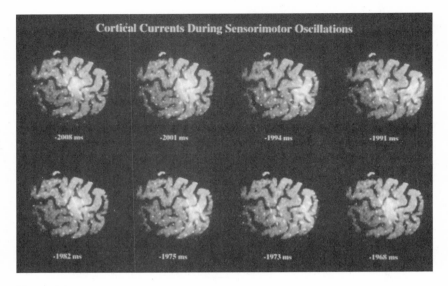

Figure 6.1
Magnetoencephalographic records (MEGs) made with multiple surface electrodes, showing temporospatial oscillations between activation of the sensory and motor regions of the cerebral cortex as the subject makes voluntary hand movements. The fourth image on the top row shows activation in both the sensory (right) and motor (left) areas of the cortex. The MEG records are superimposed on MRIs of the subject's cortex. Palest areas of those with greatest activity, surrounded by regions of lower activity. (F. Lado, U. Ribary and R. Llinás, unpublished observations.)

We should take this a step further and attempt to understand subjectivity, as it is the salient issue of this chapter. It is one thing for the nervous system to know something (the proper set of steps required for implementing digestion, for example), and quite another for *you* to know something. The issue of subjectivity is a hotly debated topic in the fields of philosophy and the cognitive sciences. But is subjectivity necessary at all? Why is it not just enough to see and react, as a robot might do? What advantage is conferred on the organism by actually experiencing something over just doing it? It is important to consider that animals may not have subjectivity but only react as if they do. Some in this field point out that because we cannot determine that animals do have subjective feelings (qualia), we can say that in fact they don't until it is demonstrated otherwise. It may be argued, however, that the burden of proof is on those who deny subjectivity in animals. For myself, I suspect that subjectivity is what the nervous system is all about, even at the most primitive levels of evolution. As an obvious corollary to that suspicion, I also suspect that consciousness as the substrate for subjectivity does not exist outside the realm of nervous system function or its nonbiological equivalent, if there is any.

We know that single-cell "animals" are capable of irritability, that is, they respond to external stimuli with organized, goal-directed behavior. It is difficult to ignore that such cellular property is probably the ancestry for the irritability and motricity displayed by sensory and muscle cells, respectively. And so we are left with the nagging feeling that irritability and subjectivity, in a very primitive sense, are properties originally *belonging to single cells.* If so, that primitive subjectivity may be built into the consciousness and subjectivity displayed by the nervous system as cells organize into the ensembles that we know as nerve cell circuits. But do take note that only certain architectures are capable of supporting and enhancing such primitive "feelings." Also note, however, that such a primitive form of subjectivity and the notion of "grandmother cells," which will be discussed further in this chapter and in chapter 10, are totally distinct concepts.

The goal of this chapter is to add further substance to the basic position of this book, namely that the issue of cognition is first and foremost an empirical problem, not a philosophical one. This issue has been addressed by some of the most distinguished biologists of this century (Crick 1994; Crick and Koch 1990; Changeux 1996; Changeux and Deheane 2000; Edelman 1992, 1993; Mountcastle 1998).

We have spoken of the embedding of universals and of the coordinate system transformations that the brain performs to do this (chapter 3). We also saw that as we trace the flow of activity into the brain (from the peripheral sensory receptors or the output organs of the body, the muscles and glands), the geometric transformations that provide functional communication between sensory and motor frames of reference become increasingly more abstract. Given this, when addressing such remote functional sites it is not surprising that terms such as "higher computational levels" have become commonplace in neuroscience. However, one may ask what is actually being computed when a neuron fires an action potential. This is not an insignificant issue. Such language implies underlying assumptions that may not apply to the brain and that may encourage misguided inquiry.

Sensory Representation

At the very forefront of brain theory is the goal of transforming knowledge relating to the properties of the nervous system into an understanding of global brain function. And so, for instance, in the study of sensory systems or pathways, we see the tendency to favor constructions that describe how cells with general sensory properties (e.g., photoreceptors) connect to cells with more specific receptive properties, and so on. The overall process, so it is supposed, is just a matter of the handing over of duty to components with successively better expertise in sensory analysis. But how can one have better expertise as one moves away from the level of direct observation provided by sensory input and into the realm of more abstract and recondite corners of brain function? Well, the fact is that reality is elaborated by brain function, and it does not come easily. The study of neurological conditions tells us that the ability to recognize reality and to respond to it may be altered in an enormous number of ways, giving us a glimpse into the amazingly cooperative nature of brain function. In this particular instance all the parts are important, even those that are silent at any particular time. As in music, in brain function silence is as important as sound.

Although this line of thinking has been central to our attempts at understanding brain function, it can also lead to misperceptions. For instance, it has lead to a belief in the appropriateness of such terms as the "face cell" or the "grandmother cell," a cell whose firing denotes the recognition or recollection of one's grandmother (see, for example, Gross and Sergent 1992; Rolls 1992). The fundamental problem with these concepts, and the line of thinking that produced them, is easily exposed. If the operation of each neuron represents knowledge of only a very specific component of reality, to whom does this information get communicated in the rest of the brain? That is, how could these neurons make themselves understood by other cells not "in the know"? What sort of cognitive deficits might we observe if such cells are damaged? Would Grandma disappear from our cognitive world if that set of cells were to die? A strong physiological argument opposing such ideas is the sobering fact that the truly galactic number of possible representations that the brain can make clearly exceeds the number of available neurons! (Tononi et al. 1992).

It is not difficult to understand how such views came about, however. In the 1950s, Wilder Penfield and Herbert Jasper made seminal contributions toward an understanding of the functional organization of the brain. Their findings were subsequently extended (inappropriately) beyond their original well-defined limit.

In those early studies (Penfield and Rasmussen 1950), patients with intractable epilepsy were treated by surgically removing the site of origin of the deleterious electrical activity. During these surgeries, in which patients were fully awake and only the scalp was anaesthetized (a painless procedure), the surgeon electrically stimulated various areas of the cortex. Within a certain cortical region, stimulation elicited muscular twitches in the fingers, toes, arms, shoulders, and so on. Similarly, in another nearby cortical area, stimulation produced sensations in various specific body parts, as reported by the patient. Through diligent work, a map of what we now call motor cortex and somatosensory cortex was constructed. Many of these cortical areas are somatotopically organized, in that the layout of the body is represented, in faithful point to point matching, by the cells of each of these cortical structures. For example, the fingers of the left hand are represented as a neuronal map of the hand (and its fingers in correct place and order) in the motor cortex for the flow of motor information to the periphery, and in the somatosensory cortex for tactile information coming from the periphery. These somatotopic mappings are distorted versions of the body, however, and for good reason. The various body parts are represented in different proportions. For instance, there are many times more neurons involved in the motor and sensory aspects of the functioning of the tongue than there are for, say, the heel. The tongue is far more articulate in all that it does than the heel. Similarly, more cortical real estate is dedicated to the skin of the index finger than is provided for a similar area of skin on the back. The tactile sensitivity of the index finger is vastly greater than that of the back, and so is its range and detail of movement. The difference in this resolution represents the order of importance to the organism: having your index finger go completely numb and useless will interfere more with your world than will numbness on a bit of your back.

If one were to draw the body as it is somatotopically represented in faithful proportion to the number of cortical cells associated with the different parts, one would have a humanoid distorted to alien dimensions. Neuroscientists refer to this map as the cortical homunculus when relating to humans.

All animals with a nervous system have a specific animunculus of one sort or another, although ours, for obvious reasons, is more neurologically "fortified" in some areas and less in others. I shall return to this issue of point-to-point spatial mapping in just a bit.

When Penfield electrically stimulated the temporal lobe of the cortex (a complicated structure that is involved with a range of functions, including auditory processing, language, and facial recognition), patients told of visual and auditory events such as "hearing a symphony" or "seeing my brother" and so on. This has led some neuroscientists to suggest that given neurons of the temporal cortex store a particular memory, as if creating a videotape of a small piece of one's life. It is not difficult to understand how such a "memory cell" theory arose; it seemed a logical next step in light of the relatively precise point to point representation of the body that was found in both the motor and somatosensory cortices.

More recently, studies have shown that cells in certain areas of the monkey inferior temporal lobe do indeed demonstrate striking response selectivity to the visual presentation of a face. Here, investigators recorded the activity of a particular neuron while the monkey was shown various pictures (see Perrett et al. 1982; Tovee et al. 1994; Abbott et al. 1996). However, these "face" cells also respond, albeit less strongly, to a variety of very dissimilar visual stimuli as well (Gross and Sergent 1992).

In studies of the neural control of primate vocalization, cells recorded in the monkey periaqueductal gray in the core of the brain stem show a clear and repeatable ramping pattern of activity prior to the vocalization. The activity begins at a set time preceding a vocalization, and reaches its peak right at the onset of the monkey's vocalization (Larson and Kistler 1984, 1986; Larson 1985; Kirzinger and Jurgens 1991, 1998; Zwirner and Jurgens 1996). Furthermore, these cells are active only preceding vo-calizations of a very specific pitch. Clearly, all we have to do is find the cells that encode for vocalizations of each and every specific pitch and we have mapped out the cells responsible for a monkey's vocalization reper-toire, right? Tempting, perhaps, but a proportion of these very specific vocalization cells also respond to general auditory stimuli and some are strikingly well correlated with eye movements of certain directions (Larson and Kistler 1984). To ignore secondary responses when inter-preting the data for a particular cell would be to misrepresent intention-ally the complexity of the system, leading to misconceptions about how it actually works.

Returning to our face or grandmother cell, findings in many systems suggest that such a categorical representation is achieved by the activity of populations of cells and not by the electrical activity of any one cell. It should be clear that the grandmother cell concept implies that the multi-ple sensory input associated with grandmother, and the multiple states that grandmother can have in real life, would make, *de facto,* such a grandmother cell a tremendous connectivity puzzle. What mechanism can one find that will bind processed information from disparate sensory sources so that, for momentary practical purposes, the resulting internal representation or sensorimotor image means the same thing? This mech-anism should also associate memories and/or thoughts with this internal construct, such as imagining/remembering a voice reading to you from the book you are holding. Just as easily you may read this book aloud, adding a definitive motor component. Yet the holding and seeing of the book, your reading aloud from it, and the fact that you may be doing so without your shoes on are all still bound seamlessly in time as a single event. Something quite different seems to be at work here than if each in-dividual neuron represented a single, predetermined, highly specific as-pect of this event. Note that in creating this experience, you are bringing together elements that are truly yours (your hand representation and your shoeless feet) and elements that are truly foreign (the contents of the book you are reading)

This raises the issue of whether the brain handles body representation in the same way that it handles the representation of objects and events it was not born with—those of the external world. Is there a single solution to the set of questions that have been posed here? Let us see.

Perceptual Unity of Consciousness—Content and Context

At the outset of this chapter we asked: Given that neurons have evolved into performing differing and specified functions capable only of representing fragments of reality, how then does the brain manage to make a singular, useful construct from these pieces? The integration of specific sensory occurrences into single percepts, or rather, the neuronal mechanisms underlying this feat, are even more amazing (and thus experimentally more challenging) when one keeps in mind that the brain does this in a context-dependent fashion. We touched on this issue in chapter 1.

The integration of specific sensory occurrences, the content of our percept, is dependent on the internal context of the brain that we generally refer to as attention (a momentary functional disposition), and is most easily recognized when comparing the functional states of wakefulness and sleep. If, while you are awake, someone whispers to you that there is a bee in your hair, you will most likely do something about it. If, on the other hand, you are asleep when they whisper, you most likely won't. If this same scenario of comparisons were under experimental conditions where it was possible to monitor the flow of auditory information from your ear into your brain, we would see that this sensory signal is transduced peripherally, in full regalia, in both circumstances (waking and sleep). Why don't you hear it when asleep? Because the signal reached only a certain stage of processing, after which point the brain ignored it—and the brain ignored it because in the sleeping state it does not incorporate sensory input into the prevailing internal context of the moment. The internal context of the brain during sleep is one that does not grant significance to the meaning of those whispered words or much of any auditory information save for the very loud (Llinás and Pare 1991). During the waking state, however, the internal context does give significance to these words, this auditory stimulus, capturing your momentary attention, if not eliciting an overt behavioral response.

The Issue of Attention

Consider the example of trying to remain attentive to a public speaker when someone seated behind you will not keep quiet. Eventually, you phase them out and only give internal significance to the words you wish to hear. I use this example because I believe it lends focus to the nuances of different internal contexts and how subtly, at a moment's notice, they may and do change. The task for the theory presented in this chapter is to suggest how the fragmented representations of individual stimulus properties observed in the primary sensory areas of the brain are linked or gathered to obtain a complete pattern (a singular percept). It is also the task of this chapter to suggest how such reconstituted patterns are given internal significance within the prevailing momentary context. We shall deal with content and context at length later in this chapter. For now, let us address the first part of the hypothesis: how it is that the brain takes the sensory-referred fragments of reality and puts them together in time as a single cognitive construct.

It has long been accepted in the world of neurological research that in humans the general circuitry of the brain present at birth is not fundamentally modified during normal maturation, but rather is only fine tuned. The neural circuitry for us to move our fingers is with us at birth; we don't have to learn this. By contrast, to play the violin, particularly with any degree of esthetic value, takes practice; this is the experiential fine tuning of synaptic connections that I spoke of in chapter 3. Both the skill and especially the musicality with which a person is able to perform a piece is clearly dependent on/limited by a complex of capabilities present at birth, but can be uncovered or facilitated to varying degrees by practice. The ability to have language, as another example, is genetically determined and thus the neuronal circuitry ascribed for this ability is with us at birth; which particular language becomes our mother tongue is the "nurture" aspect of this equation. The view and understanding of such structural *a priories* began with the identification of the cortical speech area (Broca 1861) and continued with the anatomical work of Ramón y Cajal. Cajal demonstrated that neurons were the basic units for brain organization, the "neuronal doctrine," and went on to describe the existence of well-specified neuronal circuits present in all normal brains. This functional connectivity was supported later on by Penfield's point-to-point somatotopic mapping, which applies to all normal human brains. The degree of variability observed for such point-to-point connections among humans is that which characterizes anatomical variability from person to person (height, distance between eyes, etc.), but surely having two eyes, a nose between them, and a mouth underneath is a constant that we all expect. And so a thalamus, a cortex, and the specific connectivity between them are not learned but inherited.

This structural a priori of point-to-point neuronal connectivity, referred to as "spatial mapping," is produced by the links that related neurons make with each other. Within a group of functionally related neurons there is certainly a finite number of neurons, and thus a finite number of possible connections among them. It follows that there is also a finite universe of possible representations to be created by these neurons, their connectedness, and their individual activities. However, the variations and permutations of neuronal activity with 10 billion cells in a brain are for all practical purposes limitless, especially given the human life span.

And so, we are brought to a very important question: Is it possible that the hierarchical organization produced by neuron to neuron communication is capable of putting together the shards of reality given by our senses into a single internal percept by generating all-knowing cells? The answer, as one might suspect, is probably not. A purely hierarchical connectivity alone is simply too slow and unwieldy to keep pace with the ever-changing aspects of the external world. There must be another mechanism at work.

Timeness is Consciousness

This mechanism is most likely temporal coherence. It has been stated that in brain development, "neurons that fire together wire together." A variation on this statement might be "neurons that fire together conspire together" or "timeness is consciousness." Mapping connectedness in the time domain, superimposed on top of the limited possibilities of spatial connectedness, creates a vastly larger set of possible representations through the almost infinite possibilities of combination. This is the concept of perceptual unity based on spatial and temporal conjunction. Building on physical connectivity, the nerve cells of the brain have created an "interlocking" solution: the synchronous binding in the time domain of those individual neuronal activities. By making different time-interlocking patterns, neurons can represent a unity of reality by combining the individual, fractionalized aspects of reality that each neuron carries. This time-interlocking phenomenon is temporal coherence. If whole modules of neurons (whose activities represent fractionalized aspects of the external world) electrically oscillate in phase or resonate, as we saw in chapter 2, a global activity pattern is formed. This activity pattern should have all of the components necessary for a transiently useful, internal construct of the external world in the given, present moment. And so, as an analogy, one asks how many melodies (tonal sequences) can be played on a piano. Given the permutations and combinations of simultaneously played keys, the answer is clearly in the realm of the inumerably large.

Temporal coherence is believed to be the neurological mechanism that underlies perceptual unity, the binding together or conjunction of independently derived sensory components, called "cognitive binding." It is thought to be implemented by temporal conjunction—the physiological linking in the time domain of the independently operating neural mechanisms subserving the processing of sensory and interoceptive stimuli. Similarly produced and easier to understand is "motor binding," where, as we saw with the inferior olive, motricity requires precise temporal activation of muscles in order to implement even the simplest movements correctly.

Until recently, temporal mapping in the brain has been more difficult to understand and to study than spatial mapping. This is because its study requires an understanding of the dynamics of brain function. Basically, the electroanatomy (who inhibits, or excites, whom) has been the prevailing philosophy in our studies, but it is simply not enough. Even as the concept of temporal mapping is in general becoming more accepted, in neuroscience it has been a neglected parameter. This has been so primarily for technical reasons, because it necessitates simultaneous electrical recordings from a sufficiently large number of neurons to be statistically significant. That is, one must demonstrate the simultaneity of neuronal firing by a time series analysis (e.g., cross-correlation), and this correlation must be causally linked with a sensory or motor event that it supposedly generates.

Synchronous activation of neurons that are spatially disparate is a likely mechanism to increase the efficiency of the brain. We have known for some time about such simultaneity for motricity and for motor-derived brain activity. Examples include the electrical shock produced by fish such as the electric eel or by the elasmobranch Torpedo marmorata (Bennett 1971). The "electric organ" of fish, the electroplaques (the components of the electrical whacking system) must operate at the same time. The small currents produced by each of the tiny electroplaques must sum into the electrically stunning blow these can generate by "letting go" in unison, and this requires that they activate at the same time. How is this synchronicity achieved, as the electroplaques are located at different distances from the central command nucleus? Well, the neurons in the command nucleus fire synchronously, and the conduction time (time for a neuronal signal to travel) to the electroplaques is uniform because the conduction velocities of the different motor neurons vary directly with the distance to the individual electroplaques they activate. That is to say, the axons of the motor neurons are of differing lengths; the longer axons conduct their signals faster, and the shorter axons more slowly, so the signals reach their targets, whether far or near, simultaneously. The issue here is that nature deals with the issue of simultaneity with great care, and will go the extra distance by tuning conduction velocities to assure synchronicity, without which the fish may change from a "stunner" to a "tickler." Similarly, such isochronic activation in the face of wide spatial disparity is seen in the mammalian olivocerebellar system described in chapter 2. Purkinje cells across a wide expanse of cerebellar cortex are activated synchronously by direct activation of the inferior olive (Sugihara et al. 1993; De Zeeuw et al. 1996). This is again achieved by the varying conduction velocities with the length of the input axons.

Is there evidence for synchronous neuronal activation during sensory input? This is an important issue, for if perceptual unity of objects and events of the external world is to occur through the conjunction of spatial and temporal mapping in the brain, one would expect to observe synchronous activation of neurons related to sensory input and processing—and this is what we see. In the visual system, the volley of neural activity entering the optic nerve following activation of the entire population of retinal ganglion cells is close to synchronous on to the thalamus (Stanford 1987). Stationary and moving light stimuli also evoke oscillatory responses in retinal ganglion cells that are synchronized across the nasal and temporal halves of the retina, and which evoke synchronous responses in the thalamus (Neuenschwander and Singer 1996). This means that activity from the central and peripheral aspects of the retina have similar conduction times, despite the fact that the distance the sensory axons must travel from the most peripheral ganglion cells to the thalamus may be twice that of axons arising from ganglion cells near the optic nerve. This is another case of temporal tuning to attain synchronicity.

More centrally, Wolf Singer and his colleague Charlie Gray have reported widespread synchronicity in the mammalian cerebral cortex (Eckhorn et al. 1988; Gray and Singer 1989; Gray et al. 1989). This synchronous activity from cells in a given column of the visual cortex is observed when light bars of optimal dimension, orientation, and velocity are presented. Moreover, the components of a visual stimulus that are related to a singular cognitive object (such as a line in a visual field) produce temporally coherent "gamma oscillations" (close to 40 Hz) (Gray and Singer 1989; Gray et al. 1989). These oscillations are in regions of the cortex separated by as much as 7 mm (as far as neural real estate is concerned, this is basically a different county). There is also a high correlation with 40-Hz oscillatory activity between related cortical columns. We have discussed such oscillatory resonance mechanisms before (chapter 2), when looking at the motor control signal emanating from the inferior olivary nucleus. With reference to the visual cortex, we are seeing spatially disparate ensembles of neurons whose activities are bound together in time by a distinct rhythm that oscillates at 40 Hz (Llinás et al. 1991; Nunez et al. 1992; Lutzenberger et al. 1995; Sokolov et al. 1999).

How the brain actually orchestrates simultaneity in the (neural) organization of perception in a physiological sense is as fascinating as it is complicated. Before turning to the neuronal nuts and bolts of this organizational mechanism, I would like to introduce the reader to the overt, global brain mechanism that I consider the prime candidate for implementing this essential cognitive binding event. The brain mechanism in question is as much a product of the evolutionary embedding of motricity as are the intrinsic oscillatory electrical properties of the neurons that combine to produce this mechanism.

Global 40 Hz: The Signal that Binds

Studies indicate that 40-Hz coherent neuronal activity large enough to be detected from the scalp is generated during cognitive tasks. Furthermore, some propose that this 40-Hz activity reflects the resonant properties of the thalamocortical system, which is itself endowed with intrinsic 40-Hz oscillatory activity (Llinás 1990; Llinás et al. 1991; Pedroarenas and Llinás 1998; Steriade et al. 1991; Whittington et al. 1995; Steriade and Amzica 1996; Steriade et al. 1996; Molotchnikoff and Shumikhina 1996) (figure 6.2). The 40-Hz coherent activity has been a candidate for the generation of unitary perceptual entities out of many sensory and motor vector components, which represents the details of the perceived world. What does it mean? We are confronted with a system that addresses the external world not as a slumbering machine to be awoken by the entry of sensory information, but rather as a continuously humming brain. This active brain is willing to internalize and incorporate into its intimate activity an image of the external world, but always within the context of its own existence and its own intrinsic electrical activity.

If we posit that the 40-Hz coherent waves are related to consciousness, we may conclude that consciousness is a noncontinuous event determined by simultaneity of activity in the thalamocortical system (Llinás and Pare 1991). A 40-Hz oscillation displays a high degree of spatial organization and thus may be a candidate mechanism for the production of the temporal conjunction of rhythmic activity over a large ensemble of neurons. Global temporal mapping generates cognition. The binding of sensory information into a single cognitive state is implemented through the temporal coherence of inputs from specific and nonspecific thalamic nuclei at the cortical level. This coincidence detection is the basis of temporal binding.

The Thalamocortical System and the Generation of "Self"

I have already discussed the proposition that the brain operates as a closed system: it is not surprising that the thalamic input from the cortex is far larger than from the peripheral sensory systems. This suggests that the thalamocortical iterative activity is a main mechanism of brain func-

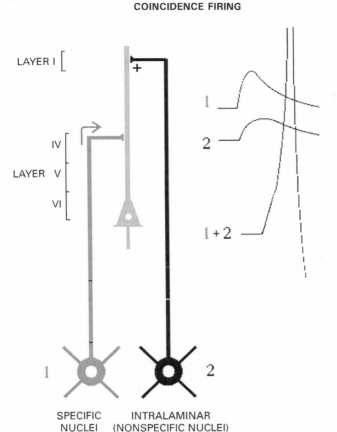

COINCIDENCE FIRING

LAYER I

IV

LAYER V

VI

1

2

1 + 2

1

2

SPECIFIC NUCLEI   INTRALAMINAR (NONSPECIFIC NUCLEI)

Figure 6.2
Simplified diagram to illustrate the generation of temporal binding due to the conjunction of coincident 40-Hz bursting activity within separate, but convergent thalamocortical pathways. Cell at left represents specific sensory or motor nuclei projecting to the cerebral cortex (layer IV), while the right hand cell represents nonspecific intralaminary nuclei projecting to the most superficial layer of the cortex (layer I). See text for details. (Adapted from Llinás et al. 1998, figure 6, p. 1847.)

tion. In addition, neurons with intrinsic oscillatory capabilities that reside in this (thalamocortical) complex synaptic network allow the brain
to self-generate dynamic oscillatory states that shape the functional
events elicited by sensory stimuli. The switching of firing modes in
thalamic neurons can trigger macroscopic changes in (global) functional
states as dramatic as the difference between sleep and arousal. In my
view, the thalamocortical system has evolved as the most efficient solution for the implementation of temporal coherence across areas of the
brain that not only subserve differing roles in reality emulation, but
which also are physically very distant from each other. How? The
thalamocortical system, by its hublike organization, allows radial communication of the thalamic nuclei with all aspects of the cortex. These
cortical regions include the sensory, motor, and associational areas. The
latter is the largest part of the cerebral cortex in *Homo sapiens*. It receives
input from the association nuclei of the thalamus and also from the sensory cortex. These areas subserve a feedforward/feedback, reverberating
flow of information.

The thalamocortical system is a close to isochronic sphere that synchronously relates the sensory-referred properties of the external world
to internally generated motivations and memories. *This temporally coherent event that binds, in the time domain, the fractured components of
external and internal reality into a single construct is what we call the
"self."* It is a convenient and exceedingly useful invention on the part of
the brain. It binds, therefore I am! Temporal coherence not only generates the self as a composite, singly perceived construct, but creates a single seat or centralization from which the predictive functions of the
brain, so critical to survival, may operate in coordinated fashion. Thus,
subjectivity or self is generated by the dialogue between the thalamus and
the cortex; or to put it in other words, *the binding events comprise the
substrate of self.*

Is the binding event actually the substrate or scaffolding of self? Following damage to the intralaminar or nonspecific thalamic nuclei (cell
groups in the thalamus that receive ascending input from a region of the
brain stem called the reticular formation), patients are not aware of the
inputs conveyed from the thalamus to the cortex by the intact specific
thalamocortical circuit (see Llinás and Pare 1991). Although inputs from

the specific thalami are received, the injured individual cannot perceive or respond to them. In essence, the individual no longer exists, from a cognitive point of view, and although specific sensory inputs to the cortex remain intact, they are completely ignored. These results argue that the "nonspecific system" is required to achieve binding; that is, to place the representation of specific sensory images into the context of ongoing activities.

Prediction Must Be Centralized—It Leads to Self

Given that prediction is the ultimate and most pervasive of all brain functions, one may ask how this function is grounded so that there evolved only one predictive organ. Intuitively, one can imagine the timing mismatches that would occur if there were more than one seat of prediction making judgement calls for a given organism's interaction with the world; it would be most disadvantageous for the head to predict one thing and the tail to predict another! For optimum efficiency it would seem that prediction must function to provide an unwavering residency and functional connectedness: it must somehow be centralized to the myriad interplays of the brain's strategies of interaction with the external world. We know this centralization of prediction as the abstraction we call the "self."

The Concept of "I"

"I" has always been the magnificent mystery; I believe, I say, I whatever. But one must understand that there is no such tangible thing. It is just a particular mental state, a generated abstract entity we refer to as "I" or "self." Consider for a moment that your brachial plexus (nerve network carrying sensory and motor innervation of the arm) is damaged. You may look at your (limp and numb) arm and say, "That's not me"—because you can't feel it. Well, it is you and yours. Somehow we have developed a strange, almost solipsistic physiological cosmology: "I only possess that which I innervate," or, "I am only that which I innervate." Odd, but perhaps that is what we actually do. So we have developed this simple rule that sort of brings together everything into one single entity we call the self. *It stands on the vestibular nucleus and pokes its head into the brain*—it has an up and a down to it, it has a visual component, a sound component, and so on.

So what is the self then? Well, it is a very important and useful construct, a complicated eigen (self) vector. It exists only as a calculated entity. Consider the following two examples of what I mean. First we have the concept of Uncle Sam. When one reads in the newspapers, "Uncle Sam bombards Belgrade," everyone understands that the U.S. Armed Forces have been deployed against that country. However, there is no such entity as Uncle Sam. It is a convenient symbol and even a convenient concept that implies existence, but it is a category without elements. The "I" of the vortex, that which we work for and suffer for, is just a convenient word that stands for as global an event as does the concept of Uncle Sam *vis à vis* the reality of a complex, heterogeneous United States. A second even more interesting example, given the decline of patriotism or the idea of "country as self," is sports advocacy. Consider the European or South American riots associated with football (soccer) matches. It is interesting to note that to such fanatical sports fans the team they root for is an extension of themselves; so much so, that, as one might do for one's loved ones or sometimes for one's ideas, they will fight and risk bodily harm defending "their team."

Secondary Qualities of the Senses as Inventions/Constructs

It should be clear that the secondary qualities of our senses such as colors, identified smells, tastes, and sounds are but inventions/constructs of an intrinsic CNS (central nervous system) semantic (c.f. Llinás 1987). This semantic allows placing sensory inputs into an internal context so that the brain may then interact with the external world in a predictive manner. As stated above, the generated abstraction called "self" is fundamentally no different from these secondary qualities of the senses; self is the invention of an intrinsic CNS semantic. It exists inside the closed system of the CNS as an attractor, a vortex without true existence other than as the common impetus of otherwise unrelated parts. It is an organizer of extrinsically and intrinsically derived percepts: the loom that weaves the relation of the organism to its internal representation of the external world.

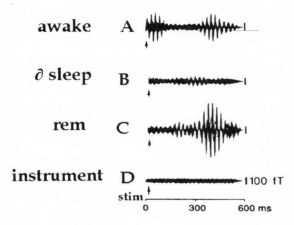

awake   A

∂ sleep   B

rem   C

instrument   D

stim

0   300   600 ms

100 fT

Figure 6.3
Oscillations in brain activity of 40 Hz recorded during sleep (δ-wave and REM sleep) and wakefulness associated with an external stimulus (bottom trace), illustrating the lack of resetting during sleep. See text for details. (Adapted from Llinás and Ribary 1993, figure 1, p. 2079.)

In actuality, however, the above philosophical discussions concerning the extent to which our perception of reality and "actual" reality overlap or match are truly of little practical importance. All that is required is that the predictive properties of the computational states generated by the brain meet the requirements for successful interactions with the external world. How this is managed by the brain, given the fractured nature of sensory input, is at the core of neurocognitive study today.

Dreaming and Wakefulness

Was it a vision, or a waking dream?
Fled is that music:—do I wake or sleep?
—John Keats, *Ode to a Nightingale*

If cognition is an intrinsically generated state, what if any distinction is there between dreaming and wakefulness? If we propose that cognition is a function of the 40-Hz thalamocortical resonance discussed above, what happens to this oscillatory rhythm during sleep, particularly dream or REM sleep? In a series of experiments, my colleague Urs Ribary and I studied the 40-Hz resonance during wakefulness and sleep, employing the technique of magnetoencephalography and using a 37-channel sensor array distributed over the scalps of five normal adults. We found that 40-Hz coherent magnetic activity was spontaneously present in the awake and in rapid-eye-movement (REM) sleep states, but greatly reduced during delta sleep (deep sleep characterized by delta waves in the electroencephalogram) (Llinás and Ribary 1993) (figure 6.3). On the other hand, and in agreement with previous studies (Ribary et al. 1991; Galambos et al. 1981; Pantev et al. 1991), an auditory stimulus produced well-defined 40-Hz oscillations in the wakefulness state, but no re-setting of the 40-Hz oscillation was observed during either delta or REM sleep (figure 6.3). There were two salient findings from these studies. One was that the waking and REM sleep states are electrically very similar with respect to the presence of 40-Hz oscillations. A second significant finding was that 40-Hz oscillations are not reset by sensory input during REM sleep, even though other studies have clearly shown that the thalamocortical system is accessible to sensory input during sleep (Llinás and Pare 1991; Steriade 1991). We consider this to be the central difference between dreaming and wakefulness: we do not perceive the external world during REM sleep because the intrinsic activity of the nervous system does not place sensory input within the context of the functional state being generated by the brain (Llinás and Pare 1991).

In more specific terms, we interpret these findings to mean that sensory input that occurs during REM sleep is not correlated temporally with ongoing thalamocortical activity (i.e., is not put into the context of thalamocortical "reality"), so it does not exist as a functionally meaningful event.

Although wakefulness and REM sleep can both generate cognitive experiences, the above findings corroborate what is commonly known, that the external environment is for the most part excluded from the imaging that is characteristic of the sleep states. In other words, it may be restated that the dreaming brain is characterized by an increased attentiveness to its intrinsic state and that external stimuli do not usually perturb this activity.

By contrast, if the responsiveness generated during the waking state is duplicated in the absence of the appropriate sensory input by virtue of activity generated via intrinsic thalamocortical interactions, then reality emulating states such as hallucinations may be generated. The implications of this proposal are of some consequence, for if consciousness is a product of thalamocortical activity, as it appears to be, it is the dialogue between the thalamus and the cortex that generates subjectivity in humans and in higher vertebrates.

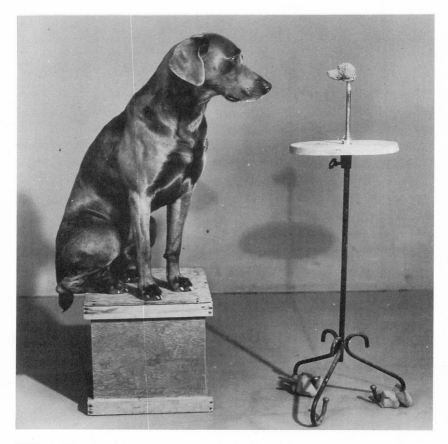

William Wegman, *Man Ray Contemplating the Bust of Man Ray,* 1978. Silver
gelatin print, 14 × 11 in.

7

Fixed Action Patterns: Automatic Brain Modules that Make Complex Movements

Complex Movements

So now we have a wondrous biological "machine" that is intrinsically capable of the global oscillatory patterns that literally *are* our thoughts, perceptions, dreams—the self and self-awareness. The next level of functional organization is again one of functional efficiency. The self, the centralization of prediction (chapters 2 and 6), cannot, however, orchestrate every feat the body must accomplish from moment to moment in the ever-changing world in which we live. Fixed action patterns (FAPs) are sets of well-defined motor patterns, ready-made "motor tapes" as it were, that when switched on produce well-defined and coordinated movements: the escape response, walking, swallowing, the prewired aspects of bird songs, and the like.

These motor patterns are called "fixed" because they are quite stereotyped and relatively unchanging not only in the individual, but in all individuals within a species. Such fixedness can be seen from the simplest to the most complex of motor patterns. For the execution of the very simple spinal reflexes, a central nervous system may not even be required. If one irritates a patch of skin on the back of a frog, a reflex to scratch is set into motion. The hind leg will swing out and up in a very stereotypical fashion, circling around to land the foot on the distressed area; this is readily repeatable and is the same across all frogs. Furthermore, this reflex may be activated and runs exactly the same in the absence of the brain and brain stem, proof that the upper central nervous system is not required for the operation of some of the more simple, rudimentary motor reflexes (Ostry et al. 1991; Schotland and Rymer 1993). In the decerebrate case above, if one impedes the trajectory of the hind leg once this reflex is activated, the hind leg will simply stop where it is obstructed from its goal. The leg will not swing out further or pull in closer to bypass the impediment, nor will it stray from its stereotypical trajectory of motion; it is quite fixed in what it can do and be. At this stage the rest of the brain would be required to intercede in order to resolve this motor impasse.

Fixed Action Patterns and the Usefulness of Stereotypical Behavior

Fixed action patterns (FAPs) are somewhat more elaborated reflexes that seem to group lower reflexes into synergies (groups of reflexes capable of more complex goal-oriented behavior) (figure 7.1). The rhythm of our walking, once initiated by the upper motor system with minor adjustments to the terrain upon which we walk, is handled largely by nervous circuitry in the spinal cord. However, it requires the activity of more than the cord to put it into context (see Bizzi et al. 1998). Neuronal networks, which specify stereotypical, often rhythmic, and relatively unchanging movements of the body when activated, are known as central pattern generators (CPGs), for this is precisely what they do. They generate the neuronal patterns of activity that drive overt FAPs such as walking (for review, see Cropper and Weiss 1996; Arshavsky et al. 1997).

We may look at FAPs as modules of motor activity that liberate the self from unnecessarily spending time and attention on every aspect of an ongoing movement, or indeed on the movement at all. Thus we find ourselves having walked miles of city sidewalks or wooded paths almost blindly while engrossed in deep conversation with a friend. Looking back on it, what tends to come to mind most is the content of the conversation and how it made us feel. Our visual memory may hold only those details of walking that required our attention, as when we perhaps stumbled briefly on a root or rock, regaining balance and resetting our gait. At such

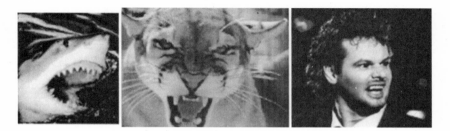

Figure 7.1
Examples of common aggressive responses in three different vertebrate species.

a moment, consciousness of what we are thinking and talking about is being briefly refocused to that of walking. That is, as a result of stumbling on the root our senses bring the focus of consciousness from the interior to the exterior, from our thoughts to our body and the world it is moving within. After changing our gait—stepping over the rock or root—walking again becomes the FAP and our consciousness goes right back to the conversation in which we were previously engrossed. This walking FAP, like all others, liberates the self to spend time and attention where it would rather be. Put quite plainly, if one had to focus on every muscle and joint and their mechanics throughout each phase of the walking cycle, consciously willing their drive, none of us would ever have those pleasant conversations through the woods on a fall day. FAPs allow us the time to do other things with our minds.

The example above also highlights another related and very important issue: the *restraining* properties of the senses on the ever-whirring thalamocortical system that we spoke of in chapter 6. In the case above, stumbling on a root momentarily brought us out of the conversation we were having. The senses remind us that there is a world outside, but we forget sometimes because the internal world generated by the intrinsic properties of the thalamocortical system can be so rich. As human beings, we differ from one another in the extent to which we pay attention to the external versus the internal world. We shall discuss that example in more depth throughout this chapter, for the restraining capabilities of the senses on the thalamocortical system also allow this system to change or finely hone FAPs as needed to interact successfully with the ever-changing world around us. But first, we must broaden our understanding of FAPs themselves—and into what amazing expressions they have evolved over the millennia.

The central nervous system is required for FAPs more complicated than locomotion, which can be elicited by the brain stem and spinal cord alone (Jankowska and Edgley 1993; Nichols 1994; Whelan 1996). The current evolutionary residence of FAPs is in the brain (see Arashavsky et al. 1997). The evolution of this process has followed the same biological imperative that we saw for the internalization of movement as the basis for mindness; in fact, it is exactly the same. The scratch reflex is purely a spinal mechanism (see Deliagina et al. 1983; Stein 1983, 1989; Mortin and Stein 1989; Jankowska and Edgley 1993). Because of its simplicity, natural selection has not found a need to move this module of function up the neuraxis and into the more sophisticated processing capabilities of the central nervous system. These capabilities are needed for more elaborate (motor) events, such as the perfectly honed, complicated finger articulations that bring to us, for instance, the beauty of Jascha Heifetz playing Tchaikovsky's *Violin Concerto in A minor.* As we watch him play this from memory, eyes closed, smiling as if far removed from his task, we wonder: a FAP? Can playing a violin concerto be a FAP? Well, not all of it, but a large portion. Indeed, the unique and at once recognizable style of play Mr. Heifetz brings to the instrument is a FAP, enriched and modulated by the specifics of the concert, generated by the voluntary motor system. We shall look further into this issue later in the chapter when we discuss the relation of FAPs to the origins of human creativity.

The Basal Ganglia as the Origin of FAPs

In the case of these more complex FAPs, it is believed that they are generated centrally by the basal ganglia (Saint-Cyr et al. 1995; Hikosaka 1998), a set of huge subcortical nuclei intimately related to the brain's motor systems (see Savander et al. 1996). For many years, neuroscience has held the basal ganglia to be the storehouse of motor programs, owing to their intrinsic circuitry. But in actuality these nuclei represent some of the least understood areas of the brain, particularly in regards to their functional organization and architecture. We know that the expression of

FAPs is supported by the interplay among a number of vastly differing parts of the nervous system and the basal ganglia (Greybiel 1995). These nuclei are localized in the center of the brain. They connect synaptically with the thalamus and receive input from both the cortex and the thalamus (for review, see Smith et al. 1998; Redgrave et al. 1999). As with the cerebellum, the majority of connections within the basal ganglia are inhibitory, with many reciprocal contacts (see Berardelli et al. 1998; Kropotov and Etlinger 1999). This is to say that neurons terminate directly on each other, so that cell A projects to cell B and B back to A, thus generating very complicated, inhibitory electrical patterns that in essence represent *the negation of activity*. If these circuits within the basal ganglia represent, when activated, the motor tapes that run FAPs, then the inactive state (momentarily *not* engaging via central and peripheral connectivity the muscle synergies that would execute and thus fully express the given FAP) is a condition of intrinsic mutual inhibition (figure 7.2). One may remember from Dante's *Inferno* a section where some of the damned souls are kept in a cauldron, but there is no demon keeping watch to make sure none of them escape their incarceration. The question arises as to why this is so. The answer is that the souls inside this cauldron are so

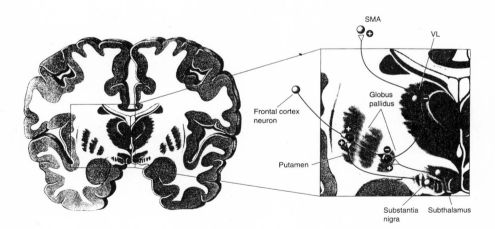

Figure 7.2
Diagram of the basal ganglia and their connections with the frontal cortex. Synapses marked with a plus (+) are excitatory; those with a minus (−) are inhibitory. (From Bear et al. 1996, figure 14.12, p. 390).

envious of one another (the sin for which they are being punished) that when one does manage to escape, the others pull him/her back in! And so the cauldron closes itself. It is the same with the basal ganglia: the intrinsic, reciprocal inhibitory activity keeps all the potential FAPs from becoming, expressing what they are supposed to be. Therefore, when a FAP is actually executed, we say that it has been "liberated" into action. The basal ganglia are the doors that when unlocked may release into action very large functions outside of the basal ganglia.

There is a wealth of neurological/physiological evidence suggesting that the basal ganglia represent or embody the neural circuitry of motor tapes. This is particularly evident if we look at the results of damage to the basal ganglia or to parts of the nervous system that heavily influence the basal ganglia (see Saint-Cyr et al. 1995; Wenk 1997; Berardelli et al. 1998). Let us take as an example a well-studied FAP, the generation of song in birds. This is particularly important here because birds sing according to their genotype (nature) and according to their phenotype (Nottebohm 1981a; Doupe and Konishi 1991; Vicario 1994; Whaling et al. 1997; MacDougal et al. 1998). Genotypically speaking, this means that a particular type of robin would have a specific song that characterizes the family. The male sings and the female recognizes the song, choosing a male on the quality of the song; but females do not sing. The ancestral song is expressed even in birds that have lost the ability to hear the sound of the song they sing. They would still sing, although the lack of auditory feedback would result eventually in abnormal song patterns (Nordeen and Nordeen 1992; Heaton et al. 1999).

This is the base song of that given species only. In normal animals this song has regional embellishments or dialects. A properly trained ornithologist can recognize the origin of a particular bird in a big city or even a particular borough by the song's signature dialect—this type of song is outer Brooklyn and not lower Manhattan. And so, in a normal bird, generic singing is modified by a learning experience when young and by the intrinsic properties of that particular animal (all brains are not exactly the same from bird to bird, for example) (Scharff and Nottebohm 1991; Nordeen and Nordeen 1993). It turns out that within a particular grouping some birds are better singers than are others, and thus have a better chance of reproduction (Tchernichovski and Nottebohm 1998). In addition to employing the brain, singing is quite a motor performance, and thus a good measure of the state of health of the animal, as well as a measure of originality of brain activity. In fact, there is brain competition, as birds will invent, copy, and steal variations of songs from each other. The songs vary in duration and complexity; the longer and the more complex, the better. Ornithologists have pieced together how a particular song is developed *before* reproduction occurs and preceding mating. They have described how song comes to fruition and maturity at mating time and then is reinvented the following year with different variations (Nottebohm 1981b; Nottebohm et al. 1986; DeVoogd 1991; Johnson and Bottjer 1993; Clayton 1997; Nordeen and Nordeen 1997; Smith et al. 1997; Mooney 1999; Iyengar et al. 1999). Next season the male will need a new song because he won't do so well with the old song. It is nature's planned obsolescence. The females recognize the males' song from last season and that that sperm may not be so good anymore! It is the same as any other champion we know of: the rise, the peak, and the fall is pervasive throughout biology. Here, a bird's rise and fall is denoted by the newness or oldness of his song (figure 7.3).

But is the song of birds actually a FAP, and how does this relate to the basal ganglia? If we look at what happens in the brain of a male bird when you remove the male hormone testosterone, we see that the basal ganglia are reduced and that in some bird species there is no song production (see Nottebohm 1980) or song production is reduced (Arnold 1975a, b). If a female, who was never meant to sing, is given testosterone, she will start singing for the first time in her life (Nottebohm and Arnold 1976; Kling and Stevenson-Hinde 1977; Nottebohm 1980; DeVoogd and Nottebohm 1981; Schlinger and Arnold 1991; Rasika et al. 1994; Nespor et al. 1996), and in bird species with singing females, females implanted with testosterone developed male-like song (Gahr and Garcia-Segura 1996)! This singing in either males or females is based on the advent of new neurons and connections within the basal ganglia (Nordeen et al. 1992; Rasika et al. 1999 for normal male development; Schlinger and Arnold 1991 for changes in females given testosterone). So, there you have a prototypical, indeed an archetypal FAP that is intrinsic in origin. This female may never have heard the song (testosterone-induced singing still happens to females raised in isolation). Yet she is fully

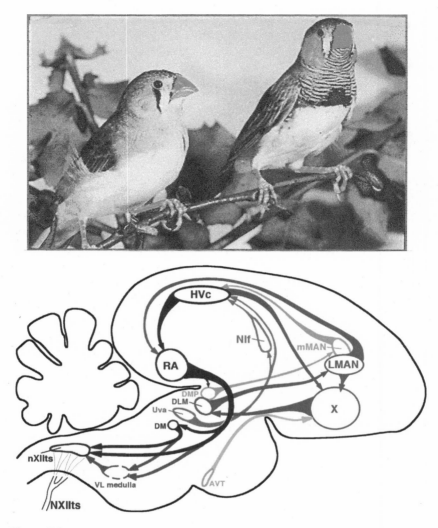

Figure 7.3

Song in birds as modifiable FAPs. (*Top*) A female (left) and male (right) zebra finch, *Taeniopygia guttata*. (*Bottom*) A schematic of a male bird's brain and song circuit, representing a sagittal section, or slice through the brain along its long axis, showing its full rostrocaudal extent. Indicated are the nuclei that form the motor pathway for song production, descending from the HVc (higher vocal center) through RA (robust nucleus of archistriatum) to nXIIts (hypoglossal nerve) and thence to the syrinx. Also shown are nuclei involved with song learning: HVc through X (area X), DLM (medial nucleus of the dorsolateral thalamus), and LMAN (lateral magnocellular nucleus of the anterior neostriatum) to RA (path not shown). Also shown: DM, dorsomedial nucleus of the intercollicular nucleus of the midbrain; Uva, uvaeform nucleus of the thalamus; Nif, interfacial nucleus of the neostriatum; AVT, ventral area of Tsai of the midbrain. HVc, RA, and X are not present in closely related species that do not produce complex vocalizations. (Diagram courtesy of Heather Williams.)

capable of generating a well-defined pattern of motricity that coordinates very specific muscle synergies that relate to the laryngeal musculature, the abdominal musculature, the intercostals, and in short the whole of the musculature necessary and sufficient to generate song. The expression of the complete FAP, the basic song of that bird's species, appears when the proper hormone is introduced. Damage to the avian basal ganglia renders both the intact male and the female given testosterone irreversibly incapable of generating normal song (Doupe and Konishi 1991; Scharff and Nottebohm 1991). And so in the case of the female, we see the liberation of an otherwise phenotypically dormant, but genotypically complete and complex FAP. This module of motor function is hardwired at birth and is activated by testosterone, naturally in the male and experimentally in the female. Just why it is that only males sing naturally and yet the FAP persists in the female is not clear; what is clear is that there is a lot of "old stuff" left around in the brain. Evidently the causal sequence that gave rise to this organization cannot easily be retraced and/or isolated in order to modify the female to eliminate an unnecessary, energetically costly component. Apparently, it is cheaper and easier just to leave it there.

Disorders of the basal ganglia provide clues to their relationship to FAPs

In the realm of human neurology, we see events that relate FAPs to the basal ganglia. Neuropathology of these nuclei may be viewed as either producing an excess of FAPs, as in Tourette's syndrome, or as a defect with the eventual loss of them, as seen in Parkinson's syndrome. In the case of people with Tourette's syndrome, where there is diagnosed partial destruction of the basal ganglia, there is an abnormal, continuous liberation of very particular types of FAPs (Coffey et al. 1994; Saint-Cyr et al. 1995; Robertson and Stern 1997; Saba et al. 1998). These patients are characterized by continuous drumming of their fingers, continuous talking, continuous arm movement, and the continuous inability to stay quiet; in a word, the typical hyperkinetic individual. These nervous, fidgety-type people are also typically quite intellectual, often athletic, and respond very quickly to sensory stimuli that relate to motricity (eye-hand coordination for example). They are witty and quick tempered; no calm or measured thought for them. All of this brings into focus the issue of automatic motor activity, how for the most part it is normally suppressed, and then subject to abnormal, involuntary liberation under very selective pathological conditions.

When terminating a motor act, or upon being stopped in the midst of an ongoing motor act, Tourette's patients are compelled by their neuropathology to *continue* the act, but may do so through the generation of words. These words are generally short, loud expletives. This involuntary continuation of motor activity works against itself. If in a crowded elevator, where for social reasons motor acts must be held in check (arm swinging, finger drumming, loud whistling), such inhibition only makes it worse for the Tourette's patient because in this case, holding back liberates! There is always a crack in the dam, so to speak, and the excess flow of water that leaks out always takes the form of curse words.

Similar to Tourette's syndrome is the affliction known as "ballism," from the word ballistic (Berardelli 1995; Yanagisawa 1996). Again, due to selective damage to specific nuclei within the basal ganglia, there is an abnormal, involuntary release of FAPs. Where Tourette's has the completion of motor activity in the form of words, ballism is characterized by spontaneously flailing the arms under similar circumstances (you may remember the strange motor affliction of Dr. Strangelove in the movie of the same name). The particular way that these syndromes manifest themselves points very clearly to certain motor activities as being modular, from an organizational and functional point of view.

Also related to the basal ganglia, but quite the opposite of what is seen in those patients with Tourette's syndrome, is that of Parkinsonism (figure 7.4). The neuropathy here is the selective degeneration of a portion of the substantia nigra, one of the nuclei of the basal ganglia (for reviews, see Colcher and Simuni 1999; Olanov and Tatton 1999). These patients are characterized by their immobile faces, dullness of thought, slow thinking—termed bradyphrenia (Kutukcu et al. 1998), quite the opposite of that seen in Tourette's syndrome—and with few, almost rangeless emotions (Benke et al. 1998). In the case of Parkinsonism, patients have extraordinary problems in moving; they have incredible difficulty in initiating any type of spontaneous or voluntary movement of even the simplest kind, such as scratching. So here we see the *lack of* abil-

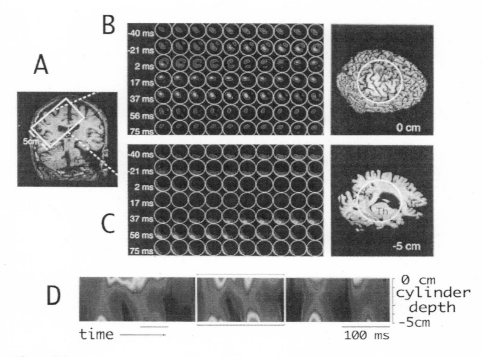

Figure 7.4

Neural basis of Parkinsonian tremor illustrated using magnetic field tomography (MFT) imaging. MFT was used to define the temporospatial distribution of cortical activity during a single resting tremor (one contraction of the flexor digitorum superficialis muscle of the hand). The results confirm rhythmic bursting in the thalamus and the sensorimotor cortex associated with tremor. For each tremor cycle, the suggested pattern of activation is as follows: Tremor is initiated 30–40 ms before muscle activation by thalamic activity. Approximately 5–10 ms later, activity is seen in the premotor cortex, followed by activation in the primary sensorimotor cortex, whose output drives the contraction of the flexor muscle, initiating the tremor. (*A*) The image at left is a coronal MRI brain slice, with the region studied (5-cm wide cylinder) indicated by a rectangle. (*B, C, left*): two sets of data, one representing recorded activity in a virtual slice at the outer edge of the 5-cm rectangle (top) and the other activity in a slice at the inner edge of the rectangle (as indicated, bottom). Each circle represents a time point. −40 ms indicates an event recorded 40 ms before muscle activation, and 2 ms indicates time elapsed after onset of muscle activation. Moving from left to right, each column represents activity associated with subsequent tremors. (*B, C right*) 3D MRI reconstructions of the regions corresponding to the outermost and innermost slice studied. Th, thalamus. (*D*) Simultaneous representation of activity pattern within the entire 5-cm cylinder over time, displayed left to right, illustrating the rhythmicity of the tremor. (From Volkmann et al., 1996, figure 6, p. 1367).

ity to release FAPs. The existence of these two syndromes, along with other motor syndromes related to disorders of the basal ganglia, suggest that FAPs are most probably implemented at the level of the basal ganglia and put into context by the reentry of the basal ganglia output into the ever-cycling thalamocortical system.

In the beginning of this chapter I said that the basal ganglia send to and receive information from the thalamus. In fact, the intralaminar complex of the thalamus (recall chapter 6) projects with a veritable vengeance onto the basal ganglia, which should suggest to the reader the idea of the physiological interplay between the self and FAPs. This is a very important issue. It is, in fact, the central issue of this chapter, and not an easy one to grasp in its full detail. So let us press on and we will get there.

FAPs and the Economizing of Choices

Having (hopefully) clarified the idea of what FAPs are, I would like to return to the issue of the intrinsic self-containment of motor programs. This intrinsic containment makes intuitive sense if we recall from chapter 2 the vast overcompleteness of the motor system. We have already seen that through the inherent architecture of this system, it may implement a given movement in an almost infinite number of ways (recall the different ways we reached for the milk carton). From a central nervous system perspective, one may ask how an animal is able to execute particular desires or goals given that those goals are often executable in a staggering number of ways. How are choices, *correct* choices, made? Clearly, making the correct motor choice can be tantamount to survival, so one suspects that, at the very least, natural selection has somehow finely polished and engrained into the nervous system a mechanism for the reduction of possible choices. Let us look into this further.

It must be understood that in theory, the nervous system can design two types of overall strategies. One is to leave the system completely free; the other is to have a built-in mechanism for the reduction of choices. By free I mean that if a gazelle sees a tiger coming, it may decide to run in a hopping fashion or with only three of four legs or to have two legs running forwards and two running backwards. The problem with a completely free system, one of almost infinite possibilities, is that if allowed to operate it would be very expensive. We know that the system is vastly overcomplete; so an efficient mechanism for the reduction of its degrees of freedom, its choices, is therefore critical. Taking too much time choosing how to escape from the tiger is not only inefficient, but also potentially lethal. A system that permits implementation of an inappropriate way of escaping the tiger, such as attempting first to make swimming motions while on land, is also ill advised and potentially lethal.

And so we see that reduction of choice is the mode of operation for which the system has been naturally selected. The motor system, given its richness, its overcompleteness, *has* to have such a global strategy for the appropriate implementation of an effective motor execution. It is simply due to the imperative of time. Of importance as it relates to FAPs, these patterns respond somewhat selectively to an urgent event in the external world requiring a well-defined, overt *strategy* such as attack and defense, finding food, reproduction, and the like, and in a timely and appropriate fashion. A set of clear constraints must be superimposed on a system that is so extraordinarily rich and predictive, and they must be very powerful. Thus birds have evolved so that they never waste time trying to fly by ineffectually beating only one wing. Of course, a bird can and will need to modify the FAP of flying once in flight, but, at the very origin of this "hardwired" FAP, as it is liberated into expression, there is the clear constraining by natural selection to do the right thing: beat both wings rather than one at activation time. That a bird is capable of flapping only one wing is obvious if one watches a bird washing itself in a bath. But this is not flying. The motor system is constrained, carved down out of its overcompleteness into (among many) this particular FAP, so that when needed it is activated at once and perfectly so.

From a physiological standpoint, the process of FAPs reduces the immense degrees of freedom of the system. In chapter 2 we spoke of muscle synergies, the co-activation of specific muscle groups in coordinated combination in order to carry out a given motor task. In that chapter, we used the example of grasping something with our hand. The beating of a bird's wings is no different: this FAP also requires the synchronous and coordinated activation of a number of different and very specific muscle synergies. Driving this motor event is the synchronous and coordinated firing of very specific motor neurons with functionally specific firing patterns, frequencies, and durations. To achieve this quite amazing feat of weeding out the extraneous, almost infinite number of other possible motor neuron activation patterns, the system has been carved by evolution's trial and error into FAPs, relatively specific modules of motor function.

FAPs Have Two Parts: Strategy and Its Implementation in Tactics

There are two *very* important aspects to this constraining of the motor system as it relates to FAPs. One is of strategy. This of course has to do with some global issue, as we have just said, a large level categorical choice such as fight or flight; one cannot do both simultaneously. But a given strategy must also be put into the context of whatever is happening at the time to the animal in the surrounding world, and so FAPs have two components. One is the strategic component as mentioned; the other is the context-dependent implementation of such strategies—the *tactics* (figure 7.5). These two components are intimately intertwined and both must be considered premotor events (chapter 2). *That* we are running from a tiger does not create the need to be doing so. The need to run comes from a sense of urgency perceived within the momentary context of the external world. Such urgency is processed within the premotor realm of prediction (I *must* run), and then the tactical solution, the appropriate FAP, is implemented: I run. Within this global decision, tactical evaluation determines that it is best to move my legs in a fashion that allows me to run my fastest. It is also strategically best to run *away* from the tiger rather than toward it. This may seem obvious, but the brain must implement every aspect correctly for survival. It is at all times a two-level decision: the appropriate strategy and the appropriate tactics within the strategy. A frog may decide to jump when the headlights come. This is clearly a good tactic, but given the number of frogs one unfortunately sees squashed on the road, the right strategy—to jump *away* from the car—is not always employed correctly or in time. Natural selection's work is never done.

It is important to clarify fully the difference between strategy and tactics as they relate to FAPs. Let us say that one is a jaguar. There is an enemy and one's strategy is to stay and fight. But *which* enemy is critical in defining the contextual tactics: fighting a snake, from a motor FAP per-

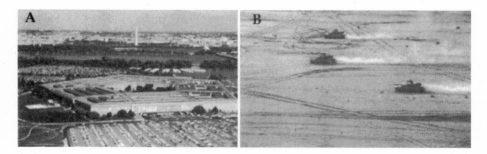

Figure 7.5
Strategy vs. tactics. (*A*) The Pentagon, headquarters of the U.S. Department of Defence, the seat of military strategy. (*B*) Marine Corps tanks; 2nd Marine Division's 2nd Tank Battalion during a tactical combined arms exercise at the Marine Corps Air Ground Combat Center, Twentynine Palms, California on February 1, 2000.

spective, is *very* different from fighting another jaguar. This two-level decision and consequent implementation of strategy and tactic holds for all creatures with a nervous system, from the most primitive to ourselves. You find yourself in a dark alley, there is trouble coming, so you begin to run and to look which way you are going to run. In this example, the strategy has already been decided. Now for the tactics: are you going to run farther down the alley or climb up the fire escape? One may look at the chosen strategy as the macroscopic event, the given implemented tactic as more the microscopic component, the fine resolution of response.

Understanding this allows us to see that FAPs must first be activated as a sequence and then the sequence put into the context of whatever is happening. It need not be as complicated as we made it for the jaguar or gazelle, or even our poor frog. The dog over there has food in front of him, but he also has an itch behind his left ear. Will he scratch first or will he eat? Clearly he cannot do both. So at all points in this type of nervous system activation, the system must opt for global events, *choosing one at the momentary expense of another, perhaps of many others.*

In a completely different physiological realm, another example is the way we examine objects of the world around us. When something calls our attention from the periphery of our visual system, we are compelled to gaze at whatever it is pulling at our attention, momentarily distracting us from our previous visual purpose. This is accomplished easily by moving our eyes, along with, in varying cases, moving our heads, necks, hips, even ankles and feet. In orienting our bodies, we get into the ballpark area of our goal. Once we are in the ballpark, we have to implement a completely different type of activity. Now we must attain the target—it is *tactical* now. In the case of eye movements, the procedure is to move the eyes so that the object of interest is shifted into the center of one's visual field and then to begin to foveate (if you happen to be a foveating animal). Foveating means switching to a higher acuity of vision, using almost exclusively the cone-type photoreceptors. In looking at something we like, such as an interesting mural, we may wish to look at this part or that part, or yet another part or area first. Here we have to decide, given our momentary level of enthusiasm, the degree of detail at which to look, for after all, looking is a subtle form of *touching*. And so again, we see the strategy, and the tactics within the strategy, at work.

The last example brings us to a crucial issue: the tedious balance between the system's deep need for an operative that greatly (and beneficially) reduces the degrees of freedom, the choices the system can make/implement, and the clearly critical need for the freedom to be able *to* make choices. This is yet a further difference between strategy and the tactics within a given strategy; it is the difference between reflexive response and volitional choice.

When something in our peripheral vision captures our attention, we move our eyes to roughly center the object in our field of vision. This is the global strategy the system adopts. It is clearly a FAP, for it is a reflex and a well constrained one; otherwise this reflex would have our eyes constantly overshooting and undershooting. Once we center this particularly fabulous painting in our field of vision, tactics now come into play: we decide which part we want to look at and foveate (figure 7.6). This tactic is *not* a FAP; it is voluntary and therefore demands conscious choice. Which part will we look at? A further and very salient point is that the tactic *inhibits* the FAP; it breaks free from its fixedness. If one corner of the painting is particularly engaging visually, I guarantee the events now in your peripheral vision will be left there. What would typically cause a reflex glance to another ballpark (strategy) has been voluntarily inhibited. Sorry, I am foveating on a given detail now.

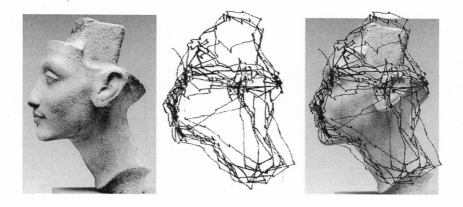

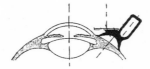

Figure 7.6
Record of eye movements (*middle*) generated in the course of examining a bust of
Nefertiti in profile (*left*). Each eye movement shown (a saccade) is volitional and
ballistic. (*Right*) Superimposition of the eye movement record over the object.
(*Bottom*) Apparatus for measuring eye movements while the head is held still.
(Adapted from Yarbus 1967; top, figure 116, p. 181; bottom, figure 13, p. 30.)

And so the system's enormous number of degrees of freedom or
choices are reduced by FAPs. At the same time, the ability to break or
modify this constraining operative, that is the ability *to* make choices—
the voluntary tactics within the given strategy—remains intact.

One last example should make this clear. You are walking on an icy
sidewalk and you slip. Your legs shoot forward from underneath you and
you are going to fall. The motor system immediately adopts a strategy
and a reflex FAP is automatically activated. At first your arms move upward and out to try to balance your body, and then they swing behind
and underneath you to break your fall. This FAP constrains the system
from operating in a completely free manner, and automatically cues up
and implements the correct compensatory response given your physical
circumstances. Natural selection has seen falling down quite a few times,
and there is no mystery as to why such a protective FAP came to be. You,

the self, haven't the time to think through and willingly drive the muscle synergies needed to invent *de novo* this protective motor event. And so natural selection saw what helps when you fall down in this fashion and over the eons honed it into a specific module that is activated by, for the most part, very specific motor circumstances: my legs are over my head and I am going *down*. FAPs are very good friends of the self.

But just how fixed are FAPs? Let's rewind the tape: you are just beginning to slip and your legs are sliding out from underneath you. But this time you are holding your mother's priceless Etruscan vase.

If the FAP that we have been speaking of were truly fixed, like that of the poor toad with the itch on his back, you would still break your fall. And, most likely, about half a second later, the vase would break too, ending its fall from where you had, as part of the damned FAP, involuntarily tossed it into the air.

But the vase *is* priceless, and what's more it belongs to your mother. The FAP does not know this, but you do. The FAP notwithstanding, we know exactly what the true outcome of this situation is likely to be. You fall straight on your duff and the vase, still in your hands and probably centered on your lap, is fine.

So what happened? Did the "appropriate" FAP *not* get released/activated? It most certainly did—as I said before, this is automatic, very fast. Ah, but so are the predictive properties of the brain. And your slipping and falling is nothing new to the thalamocortical system, either (remember from chapter 3 I said that we must move within the world in order to embed?), so predicting the consequences is both easy and automatic. There is the predictive sensorimotor image: if I break my fall, the vase will shatter into a million pieces. The voluntary solution? Don't break the fall. That is, tactically inhibit the FAP, don't let it run its stereotypical course, consciously override it: hold on to that vase at all costs! If you are not convinced that the FAP that helps you break your fall is not activated first and then overridden, just recall similar situations you have been in, and the difficulty of adjusting through the fall—to hold on to that vase or cup of coffee.

Let us briefly review. We have a motor system that when driven by global strategies implements contextually appropriate FAPs; the appropriateness comes from the immediate reduction of possible choices by the given strategy the system adopts. These FAPs are relatively hard wired at their origin and so may be considered as reflex at the time they are activated. As modules of automatic motor function, they have been formed and honed by evolution to save (computational) time as an efficient antidote to a vastly overcomplete motor system; with their timeliness of contextual activation and their dependability of execution, FAPs thus save time for the self, the seat of prediction. Once activated, however, most FAPs may be tactically modified from their stereotypical motor expression, as the given context requires. This "breaking out" or overriding of a given motor event that is constrained by the FAP being executed is accomplished by the thalamocortical system, the self, making volitional choices that arise from weighing the information and predicting consequences of the unfolding context of the given situation. It is the necessary advent of consciousness to an otherwise responsively fixed repertoire of movement.

Language as a Premotor FAP

To conclude this chapter, I would like to touch on something we will handle more fully in chapter 10, but for very different reasons. We can learn something very interesting from the Tourette's Syndrome we talked of earlier. It is worthwhile to note that the clear symptoms of Tourette's occur across people of *all* languages; this suggests something very fascinating about how the organization of the brain subserves language itself. That is, that language itself is a FAP. It is a premotor FAP at that, and most likely very intimately related to the activity of the basal ganglia, as suggested by the clinical symptoms of at least one patient whom I have seen and reported on in a collaborative study entitled "Words without Mind" (Schiff et al. 1999). This study was conducted with my colleagues Fred Plum and Nicholas Schiff, distinguished neurologists from Cornell Medical School, and my friend and collaborator Urs Ribary, who is, as I am, from NYU Medical School. In the patient studied, a massive stroke had left almost nothing functional save for the basal ganglia and a part of the cortex known as Broca's area. This area is responsible for the generation or motor aspects of language. The stroke also left intact parts of the

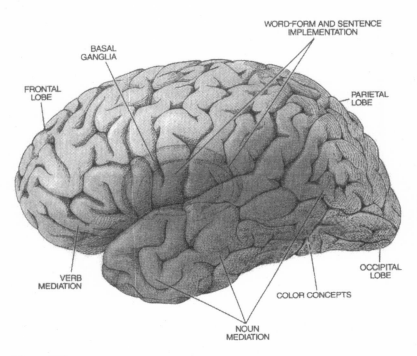

BASAL
GANGLIA

WORD-FORM AND SENTENCE
IMPLEMENTATION

FRONTAL
LOBE

PARIETAL
LOBE

OCCIPITAL
LOBE

VERB
MEDIATION

COLOR CONCEPTS

NOUN
MEDIATION

Figure 7.7
Language centers of the brain. The left hemisphere comprises word and sentence implementation structures and mediation structure for various lexical items and grammar. The collections of neural structures that represent the concepts themselves are distributed across both right and left hemispheres in many sensory and motor regions. (From Damasio and Damasio, 1992, p. 92.)

thalamus in such a way that these parts, along with the basal ganglia and the cortical Broca's area, shared some interconnected circuitry between them. This person is in a coma and has been so for the last 20 years, and every measurement performed objectively and by means of noninvasive imaging has indicated that most of this patient's brain is functionally dead. And yet this person, in a vegetative state, will occasionally generate words (figure 7.7).

So here we have someone who has lost all other abilities and the only ability left intact is the ability to generate words. This again reaffirms that the nervous system appears very much to be organized in functional modules. In this case, word generation is an intrinsic property of the brain. This circumstance, the random emitting of words with no consciousness behind the FAP that produced them, is very sad. However, the opposite and equally possible scenario is perhaps more harrowing: if you damage the system, the individual may be capable of understanding language, of understanding prosody, of seeing and hearing and interacting with the external world, except that he/she will be incapable of generating words. But again, the point here is that these cases clearly point to a modular organization of function in the nervous system.

FAPs are subject to modification; they can be learned, remembered, and perfected. How does the brain learn and remember anything? The self? We shall look into these issues in chapter 9.

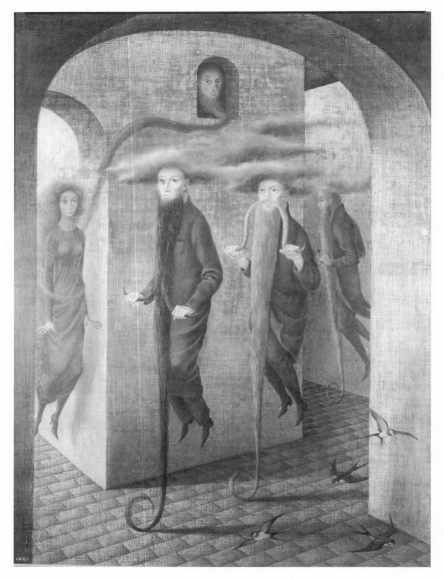

R. Varo, *Capillar Locomotion*, 1959. Oleo/masonite, 83 × 61 cm.

8

Emotions as FAPs KEY CHAPTER, READ AGAIN!

It is always healthy to approach the issue of emotions with a good measure of trepidation. There are few topics of inquiry as thorny as our affective world. The fact that emotions are for the most part irrational, and that they can enslave our rationality (according to Hume) is probably at the root of their thorniness. On the plus side, they are the reason for our wanting to survive, and our inspiration. Indeed, the properties and vicissitudes of our emotional selves are often referred to as our "humanity." These issues have a long and distinguished history, with misunderstanding of human motive at its helm. The "face that launched a thousand ships" in Homer's legendary *Iliad* is a case in point. It was not only the face, nor probably any of Helen's other anatomical characteristics that mobilized Agamemnon's armada against Troy. The main culprit most probably was the loss of love, injured pride.

So how shall we address such a complex topic? I propose that we consider that emotions are elements in the class of "fixed action patterns," or FAPs, where the actions are not motor but premotor. Further, we may consider that, as with muscle tone that serves as the basic platform for the execution of our movements, emotions represent the premotor platform as either drives or deterrents for most of our actions. However, unlike muscle tone where the level of muscle activation is the parameter regulated, emotions are notorious for their variety.

Reflecting on the history of humanity we find emotional states well characterized in the Western, Judeo-Christian tradition in the form of "the cardinal Sins" (pride, rage, greed, lust, envy, sloth, and gluttony) and the somewhat lesser known and not easily reconciled with true emotional states, the "cardinal Virtues" (justice, prudence, temperance, fortitude, faith, charity, and hope). According to a modern dictum the latter seven have the quality of being their own reward (truly intrinsic), an idea that may derive from, or at least reflect, practical needs surrounding the origins of settled, agricultural society—in essence, the notion of "enlightened self-interest."

That issue aside, emotions in general are among the very oldest of our brain properties. They are enacted by the rhinencephalon (see Velasco et al. 1988, 1989), whose activity supports and generates not only our emotional feelings, but also a host of motor, autonomic, and endocrine postures that probably evolved as states of readiness to action, as well as modes of social signaling of intentionality. From a neuroscience point of view the question of the neurological basis for our affective world is the topic of classical and contemporary research (Brown and Schafer 1888; Bard 1928; Kluver and Bucy 1939; Hess and Rugger 1943; Hess 1957; Weiszcrantz 1956; Hunsperger 1956; Fernandez de Molina and Hunsperger 1959, 1962; Downer 1961; Geschwind 1965; Fernandez de Molina 1991; Damasio 1994, 1999; LeDoux 1996, 1998; Rolls 1999). One would not be surprised if emotional states were to be simple stereotypical responses; the cardinal entities (in particular the sins) may be triggered by peptide modulators to the point that the universal characterization may be recognized by most human cultures.

Sensations Are Intrinsic Events and Emotions, Global Sensation FAPs

The relationship of emotional states to actions, and indeed to motricity, is all important, for under normal conditions it is an emotional state that provides the trigger and internal context for action. But the underlying emotional state, the "premotor FAP," does not only trigger the action as a FAP; it is also expressed in the form of another accompanying motor

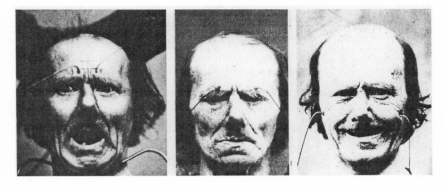

Figure 8.1
Examples of facial expressions generated by the selective stimulation of different combinations of muscles in the face. (From Duchenne de Boulogne 1862 [republished 1990] plates 13, 31, 65.)

FAP (such as a facial expression), which telegraphs to others the context (motivation) for the action and possibly the imminence of the action itself. Examples of such motor patterns can be artificially generated by electrical stimulation of the motor nerve branches in the face, without the emotional content (figure 8.1). If one inadvertently touches a very hot pan on the stove, the rapid pulling back of the hand (a FAP) is generally preceded and accompanied by a grimace (a motor FAP) and an outburst (another motor FAP) (Darwin 1872). As with other FAPs, however, the expression of an emotional state can be and often is suppressed. G. Gordon Liddy, of Watergate fame and more recently a radio talk-show host, used to impress people at Washington parties by holding his hand over a flame. "What's the trick?" someone once asked. "Not minding" he replied.

One need not invoke the very sophisticated emotional world of humans to see the inextricable relationship between emotion and action, for even the motor FAPs of relatively primitive animals are accompanied by a well-defined emotional component. This emotive element is also related to the issue of "qualia," which we shall discuss in detail a few chapters from now.

In order for a motor FAP to be generated, the input that triggers it must be amplified and put into context some time *before* the FAP is activated. There's a fire! Run! It makes intuitive sense as well; one does not want to

★ INDIVIDUAL INSTANCES OF SUBJECTIVE CONSCIOUS EXPERIENCE, WHAT IT FEELS LIKE, EXPERIENTIALLY,

just start triggering FAPs without good reason. But the input that activates a FAP need not be so alarming. It may be as simple as an itch, which for the most part is a very small stimulus. Small indeed, if one considers that *all* of one's skin is innervated and thus generating background activity almost continuously from all over the surface of the body. Now the skin is one of the largest organs in the body, and yet we react aggressively to a mosquito bite by slapping ourselves in an attempt to kill the offender. Input, in the form of sound or the small sting, generates a brief emotional reaction and thus a motor FAP, the slap, is activated. If it happens to be a spider crawling on you and you have a bit of arachnophobia, well, there goes your mother's vase! Something as insignificant as a mosquito bite or a spider wandering over your surface may evoke not just a sensory response, but actually a brief emotional state. Even a benign itch, as those who have spent time with a limb in a cast will know, can be amplified to cause maniacal behavior. We will go to any length to stop the itch, sticking anything we can find down inside the cast to that wicked place our fingers cannot reach. And when we simply can't reach the spot that itches, an even larger emotional state may be unleashed. What we understand from this situation (wearing a cast) is the importance of this kind of amplification of sensory input into an emotional state, for emotional states set clear contexts for and from which the thalamocortical system may operate.

So what do we mean by an "emotional state"? Well, I would like to relate such states to non-motor FAPs and beyond, as we shall see. Let's begin by agreeing that emotional states give context to motor behavior. In this sense, both pain and the next step, fear, are emotional states. The reader may believe that the feeling of pain relates to given emotional states, but is pain itself an emotional state? I would argue that yes, it is. A person who has a malfunctioning frontal lobe in the cerebral cortex, say in the cingulate cortex (Brodmann's area 24), can receive a sensation that activates specialized pain (nociceptive) brain pathways, but the activation of the pathways will not generate pain (see Devinsky et al. 1995; Kuroda et al. 1995; Sierra and Berrios 1998; Heilman and Gillmore 1998). The patient may recognize that the stimulus should lead to pain, but it is also clear to him that the sensation is not stressful in the way we typically know "pain" to be. If you ask, the person may say, "Yes, I feel the pain but it doesn't hurt." This is, however, not the usual response to a painful stimulus. You may want to use the argument that they are separable to support the view that pain and the emotion it generates are separate events. Well, that would be so if by pain we mean the purely sensory experience and not the unpleasantness associated with pain. Most of us actually consider the unpleasantness the pain, and not whatever else was associated with it. "It hurt like hell, and I also felt the squeezing of the thumb as the hammer hit it?"

The cingulate is activated mostly when you are in pain of the intractable, long-term type, such as that from cancer (Devinsky et al. 1995; Rainville et al. 1997; Casey 1999) (figure 8.2). Interestingly, the cingulate cortex is also activated when one makes an *error*. Oh no! Not the vase! When you think of it, a mistake or error or oversight leads to a pain of sorts, certainly a distinct emotional state that we all know only too well. Very importantly, it is a pain that is not *localizable* but nevertheless is very profound, as profound as the feeling of pain we feel when those we care for are hurt or in distress. Related to this is a similar form of "deep pain" described by psychiatric patients; whether one can call it "psychological pain" or not, it is often the reason why many of these patients commit suicide. The issue is that it is not localizable. In fact, no pain is localizable. The cutting of a finger and the pain it brings seems localized, but it is simply a co-activation of pain, the emotional state, and general tactile stimulation. The unpleasantness of pain is an emotional state generated by the brain (Tolle et al. 1999; Treede et al. 1999), not an event that somehow resides at a particular body location (Greenfield 1995).

Let's put it this way. The peripheral receptors and their neural pathways leading to the central perception of pain, that is, to the sensation, define the process underlying the generation of pain (figure 8.2). Sensations are intrinsic events, a product of the ongoing activity of the nervous system that finds a way onto the stage of consciousness. Sensations are *truly intrinsic,* in that they can also be attained or obtained in the *absence* of activation of sensory pathways. During dreaming we feel many different sensations (Zadra et al. 1998), yet none of the things we feel in our dreams comes via the pathways that convey such sensations during the waking state. You will remember from chapter 6 that although these sensory pathways are capable of transducing stimuli from the external

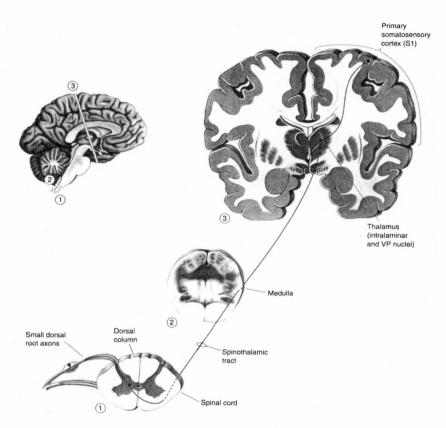

Figure 8.2
The spinothalamic pathway for the perception of pain. The pain input is conveyed from the spinal cord up the neuraxis to the thalamus, and thence to the primary somatosensory cortex. See text for details. (From Bear et al. 1996, figure 12.16, p. 328.)

world, the activity of these pathways is not given significance by the cycling thalamocortical system during dream sleep. And so, the sensations we feel during the course of a dream are a complete confabulation on the part of our brain. They derive from the activation of different thalamocortical sectors as it creates the dream world while we sleep. The sensations that we feel during dreams are so because they are constructed and placed into the context of the dream. If someone is talking to you in the dream, you will hear words; if you are falling into a steep chasm in your dream, you will feel as if you are falling. Yet your body is actually undisturbed and unmoving, asleep in your bed. Further proof that sensations are an intrinsic event of the nervous system comes from the fact that we may fly in our dreams, with arms outstretched or at our sides. This experience may come complete with full sensations of swooping, gliding, and hovering, feeling the wind and chill as we fly, and even the rain in our face. To fly unaided is something that very few of us have ever actually felt in waking reality through our bodies, *through the activation of our sensory pathways*. So in thinking on these matters, it may be a good idea to separate the carriers of sensory activity from the actual executors of sensation.

The sensory pathways do not execute sensations; they only serve to inform the internal context about the external world; during dream sleep they do not even do this. In both states, sensation is a construct given by the intrinsic activity of the brain, within the momentary internal context given by the thalamocortical system.

In this regard, we may look at emotions as the *global sensation* aspect of FAPs, if not as the FAPs themselves. They are clearly different from the motor aspect of FAPs but are nonetheless intimately related; they are often inseparable at both the intuitive and the physiological level. Emotions relate very clearly to areas distinct from the basal ganglia but nonetheless closely associated with them (Saper 1996; Heilman and Gilmore 1998). Emotions are linked to the motor aspects of FAPs (the workings of the basal ganglia) by access through the amygdala and the hypothalamus and their associated connectivity with the brain stem (Bernard et al. 1996; Beckmans and Michiels 1996). Though they are intimately related, I shall address the hypothalamus (or hypothalamic complex, for it is a group of related nuclei) and the amygdala (or amygdaloid complex, also a collective of related nuclei) separately.

FAPs and the Generation of Emotional States

The Hypothalamus

Today it is well established that the FAPs that are related to vegetative and emotional events are triggered by hypothalamic activation. The hypothalamus is a key structure in the generation of emotions *and* the vegetative and endocrine activities of the body. This is important because the FAPs that generally accompany emotional states require that the nervous system, in addition to generating coordinated motion, must also modify other parameters/systems of the body (see Spyer 1989 for review). Thus, when a bird is threatened and it must respond with flight, the rapid, synchronized activation of the chest muscles necessary for the generation of winged force is preceded slightly by an enormous increase in blood flow to those muscles. Without this increase in local circulation, the muscles would not have available the oxygen necessary to sustain the increased contractile force, and the animal would not be able to overcome inertia and become airborne. There is likewise a commensurate increase in heart output and respiratory activity (an ongoing motor FAP itself!) just before the actual execution of the motor FAP that we somewhat glibly recognize as flying. And so we see that the generation of a motor FAP is accompanied by an equally complicated and well-orchestrated control and activation of many body functions that are required to successfully execute a given FAP.

The hypothalamus is the system that regulates, as a master switch, the generation of all of these components without which the motor or the cognitive component, the conscious, *emotional* component, of the response could not be triggered (Sudakov 1997) (figure 8.3). The hypothalamus provides the physiological link between the emotional state—in the bird's case fear—and the motor FAP that is the appropriate response: flight.

Now in the case of animals where the amygdala has been lesioned (Weiskrantz 1956) or the forebrain is damaged but the hypothalamus is left intact, motor FAPs accompanied by what we would clearly recognize as emotional expression may be activated. Experimental stimulation of certain areas of the hypothalamus produces a response that appears as rage (see Smith and deVito 1984; Schwartz-Giblin and Pfaff 1985–86). This rage is, however, termed "sham" if the brain is not fully intact. Such emotional display is only the outward manifestation of what we associate in our minds with particular internal/emotional states—but the actual context of this state is absent (a bit like the issue illustrated in figure 8.1). The animal may produce the sounds and gestures associated with what we recognize as fear or pain or rage, such as hissing and the showing of

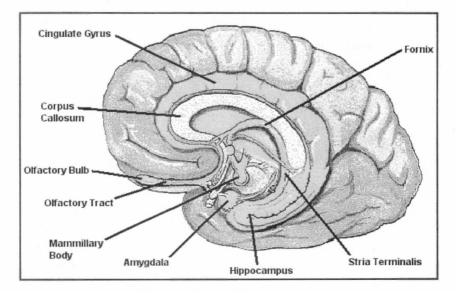

Figure 8.3
Diagram of the brain regions making up the limbic system, including olfactory bulb and tract, hypothalamus (mammillary body indicated here is part of the hypothalamus), and hippocampus. See text for more details. (From PSYweb.com.)

teeth, but in the sham condition. These sounds and gestures are emitted in the absence of the emotional state, the context that normally generates these outward manifestations. Similarly, sham emotion is also present in humans, such as when someone sheds tears of the crocodile variety. Actors learn to weep like that. And so again we see that emotions, like their motor counterpart, are FAPs in their own right. They are associated with the motor counterpart, but the above points to their somewhat clean and complete removal, implying that they are in fact discrete physiological entities.

The Amygdala

From the above discussion it follows that we should ask, "Where does the neuronal substrate for feeling emotions, as opposed to their outward manifestation, reside?" Experimental activation of the amygdala (fig. 8.3) by electrical stimulation (Fernandez de Molina and Hunsperger 1959; Velasco et al. 1989) or application of excitatory amino acid transmitters in animals elicits physiological and behavioral signs consistent with the emotional states of fear and/or distress (see LeDoux 1998). Long-term stimulation of the amygdala produces stress-related illnesses such as gastric ulcers (Morrow et al. 1993; Ray et al. 1993). We see the same in human beings who have abnormal activity in this nucleus due to epilepsy. This abnormal activity is clearly correlated with the feeling of emotional content but without the correct or appropriate context, as in being very frightened when there is nothing to be frightened about (Charney and Deutch 1996).

Likewise, lesions of this nucleus will produce the well-known Klüver-Bucy syndrome (Klüver and Bucy 1939; Weiskrantz 1956; see for reviews Horel et al. 1975; Trimble et al. 1997; Hayman et al. 1998), in which animals (and humans as well) are unusually placid and emotionally unengaged. Animals or humans with damage to the amygdala are typically unable to muster the vehemence required for the initiation and completion of even the simplest of acts. They also seem incapable of generating the general emotional feelings that normally accompany threatening or even painful situations. Perhaps even more interesting, Klüver-Bucy individuals are also unable to recognize the context of danger even though otherwise unimpaired from a sensory or motor perspective. Outwardly, this appears very similar to the Parkinson condition we spoke of earlier. But neurologically, the origin of these outward symptoms is very different. A Parkinson patient cannot express the emotional state because their associated motor FAPs are no longer physiologically accessible; the Klüver-Bucy patient has the motor FAPs available but not the emotional or contextual amplification necessary to liberate these FAPs into expression. In a classic paper on this subject, the issue of the "disconnection syndrome" postulated by Geschwind (1965), deafferentation of amygdalar input from the cortex resulted in an inability to trigger either the forward amygdalar activation pattern toward the thalamus, responsible for engendering the cognitive component, or the down going input to the hypothalamus, medial gray substance of the brain stem or the pons and medulla, which are responsible for the motor expression of emotions (Fernandez de Molina and Hunsperger 1962). Disconnection syndrome became the accepted view, as it could explain experiments such as those of Downer (1961), who showed that damage to the connectivity between visual cortex and amygdala, while not producing blindness or other visual impairments, resulted in a modality specific Klüver-Bucy syndrome—that is, in the inability to generate emotional conditions by visual stimuli but not via other sensory inputs.

The Rhinencephalon

Associated with the amygdala is a set of cortical regions collectively known as the rhinencephalon; these are believed to have evolved from the olfactory system. This rhinencephalic system primarily consists of the part of the brain that directly surrounds the basal ganglia. This "circle" contains the olfactory epithelium and olfactory bulb, the cortex immediately behind the olfactory bulb called the pre-piriform cortex, the piriform cortex itself (so named because it is shaped like a pear), as well as the entorhinal cortex and the hippocampus. In front of this structure is the cingulate that we have already talked about. All of these areas seem to be deeply related to the feelings of emotions and the activation or release of FAPs, once the emotional functional states are contextually instated. The activity of the cingulate cortex is of special interest because damage to this structure may interfere with the feeling of pain and other emotional components (Rainville et al. 1997). This part of the cortex is deeply related to emotions by means of its connectivity with the amygdala, as well as the thalamus, basal ganglia, and hypothalamus. These interconnections form the neuronal bases for the acquisition and motor expression of emotional states (See Adrianov 1996; Saper 1996; Heilman and Gilmore 1998; Davis 1998).

Olfaction and Emotion

From the above, the reader may be wondering what olfaction—the sense of smell—has to do with emotion. In human beings, the olfactory system, compared with vision or hearing, offers a rather limited amount of information about the external world. Of course, we recognize quite a large number of odoriferous substances, but the categorizations that mostly come to mind are very global and simple: is it a pleasant smell or an unpleasant one? Precious little else is noticed, unless one happens to be a wine connoisseur, a superb cook, or a perfume chemist. It is probably this type of grossly divided and categorized experience—yea or nay—that most clearly describes what consciousness would be for very primitive animals. But here again we see the macroscopic strategy of the brain, the reduction of choice: this smells awful, so don't eat it. This smells right, mate with it (Doty 1986; Shipley et al. 1996). This mechanism is clunky, big, overseeing, and seemingly not very vast in scope—and on the other hand extraordinarily powerful for smells very closely linked to emotional states that release the appropriate motor FAPs necessary for survival. Even animals who have an olfactory apparatus as exquisite as that of bloodhounds seem to use olfaction as a "go to" or "away from" cue, in spite of all the clues they are given to make more refined evaluations. This may be the product of what is being measured. Olfaction analyzes the chemistry of things; that is, it is a molecular probe and as such can say very little about the macroscopic nature of things, unlike touch or sight.

Although "this smells right, mate with it" sounds a bit crude, it is also to a large extent how things happen for most species. As interesting as this attracting ability is, the issue of olfaction (figure 8.3) being related to emotion brings to light a very thorny issue that is strongly debated at this time. It is the issue of sensory inputs that may deeply modify our behavior without those inputs ever reaching the level of consciousness. At present, the topic of the vomeronasal system in humans (influence of pheromones) carries much weight in discussions about consciousness. There have been clearly questionable suggestions, given the lack of central connectivity of this vestigial sensory system, that this secondary olfactory system may activate attitudes of like or dislike between people. Furthermore, it apparently does so without reaching consciousness. In other words, the information driving such decisions has arisen from a peripheral receptor organ located in the anterior part of the nose that is responsive to pheromones. According to such views, we may find ourselves quite attracted to or repelled by someone without so much as seeing or talking to that person.

A more likely scenario to explain irrational likes and dislikes is that other "subliminal" inputs are responsible. It is unquestionable that certain attitudes or emotional states of like or dislike may be implemented long before the inquisitive power of consciousness. The well-known seventeenth century verse by Thomas Brown about his teacher John Fell, bishop of Oxford, puts it succinctly.

I do not love thee Dr. Fell
The reason why I cannot tell
But this I know and know full well
I do not love thee Dr. Fell

This raises a very important issue, for it relates to the possibility that behavior, in its incredible range of detail and expression, may be deeply modulated by physiological events that are not experienced at a conscious level. These events nonetheless exert a deep influence on the ultimate goals implemented by the thalamocortical system at any given time, and it may be that some animals operate *only* in this mode. That is, if the system is properly organized, the proper behavioral response to incoming stimuli may simply not require consciousness.

Let us think about this for a moment. Under consideration is the hypothesis that certain attitudes and intentions are related to subconsciously received stimuli. Some behavior is subconsciously activated, but slow in expressing itself; this system does not have the immediacy to address stimuli requiring more urgent action, such as reacting to a hard object flying straight at you. Thus, the emotional states engendered by this system may be analogous to the feelings of well-being that we experience after having a meal, where most of the ingestive steps are treated by the nervous system as not requiring the intervention of the conscious self.

What does this say about consciousness? It tells us that consciousness really represents the solution for an over complete system, very much like FAPs. If FAPs represent modules of fleeting but well-defined function within the motor domain, used and forgotten as needed, consciousness represents a similar module of function, but one of *focus*, also fleeting, utilized within the context of the moment and discarded. Again we see the reduction of choice, choice of where focus is best used, because we cannot focus on everything that is continuously occurring inside and outside of our bodies. The physiological events that operate over longer time frames, such as the vegetative functions of digestion or wound healing, for the most part don't reach consciousness because they don't require its predictive, decision-making properties. Consciousness is discontinuous; global strategies of focus mandate that it must be so.

Consciousness and Emotions

In terms of FAPs and the emotional states that are associated with their liberation, there is a glimmer here of something very interesting and very different. Although the thalamocortical system is capable of activating cognition and consciousness, cognition and consciousness *probably evolved from the emotional states that trigger FAPs.*

As we have discussed, the thalamocortical system is extraordinarily rich in its predictive capabilities. In order for the system to be able to make a decision once prediction has occurred, the system must be able to focus on what are probably the best solutions to the problem, on reduction of choice. What I am going to do about this prediction defines my strategy, and the execution of the solution defines the tactics or FAPs. Strategy is the reduction of choice, the quick entrance into the right ballpark. Do you like it or not? Will you attack or defend? It is what we all do at one level or another before we act (execute a given movement). The important point here is that the system has to decide which overall strategy is going to be implemented. One strategy will always supplant the other; the system is organized to prioritize momentary emotional states, choose one as the most important, and then act on it.

Consider this example: two individuals get into an argument and are about to kill each other, but something unexpected happens that is so funny that they both cannot help but laugh aloud. In an instant this melts away all of the strategic implementation that would have been war; it is an entirely different strategic operative now. Strategy is an either/or construct. Will the dog scratch the itch or eat his food? One or the other but never both. Given the complexity of the decisions and the speed at which the nervous system must implement a given global strategy, the only solution that will make this work is one in which the animal is *conscious* of the particular emotional state. Why? Because consciousness has the great ability to *focus*—this is why consciousness is necessary. It is necessary because it underlies our ability to *choose.*

The reduction of all possible choices to a useful set of the most probable solutions for the particular situation is a necessary prerequisite to effective behavior. The strategy of reducing choice by picking any solution, regardless of its potential feasibility just to save time, is counterproductive, so natural selection has weeded it out. Another example: what if the control panel of a modern fighter jet had, instead of all those complicated instruments, a little face that tells you how everything is, at that moment, by its *expression?* You are in a heated battle; there is no way that you would be able to look at every instrument and gauge under such conditions. So you have a face—if the face is smiling, it means "Do what you must! Don't worry about the condition of the plane, you don't have time!" You need an apparatus that can direct one to focus and choose— and that *is* consciousness! The face is transforming all the incoming information into one coherent event. Because operating from a single event is always easier, it is far more powerful than continuously having to take into consideration an ever changing set of variables within an ever changing point of governance. This is why there is but one seat of prediction, *and thus consciousness.* A system with only one or two possible states would not require consciousness. The issue of over-completeness then becomes absolutely central, as is the issue of the speed of execution, from both the perceptual and motor points of view.

So what we have is a system that has evolved to be able to acquire inputs, to put those inputs into the context of what is going on internally and into the context of what is going on externally (chapter 3). But how do we combine FAPs, emotions, and consciousness into one directed output? As I said earlier, the thalamocortical system, especially the nonspecific intralaminar system, projects extremely aggressively to the basal ganglia— and thus, as expected, there is no perception that is ever separated from a possible, functional, motor implementation.

In chapter 7 I spoke of Jascha Heifetz and the complicated repertoire of fingering articulations necessary to play the violin at such a level of proficiency (or to play the violin at all). Although it seems intuitively impossible that something as complicated and exacting in detail as the finger movements involved in playing Tchaikovsky's *Violin Concerto* would be a FAP, it is an automatic module of discrete motor function. It must be. Think of it this way. When a soloist such as Heifetz plays with a symphony orchestra accompanying him, by convention the concerto is played purely from memory. Such playing implies that this highly specific motor pattern is stored somewhere and subsequently released at the time the curtain goes up. It also says something about the rich emotional state the soloist must be in, to be able to focus on, to release into expression a FAP as complicated and lovely. From this example it is evident that a FAP can be learned. Better still, a human FAP can be modified by experience (Graybiel 1995).

Let me pursue this further. There are and will be other great violinists, but Jascha Heifetz was a unique talent. Can we speak of such talent scientifically? Can the issue of human creativity be put into biological terms? Yes, I believe so. And whereas we can talk quite rationally about creativity and the human brain, the neural processes underlying that which we call creativity have nothing to do with rationality. That is to say, if we look at how the brain generates creativity, we will see that it is not a rational process at all; creativity is not born out of reasoning.

Let us think again of our motor tapes in the basal ganglia. I should like to suggest to you that these nuclei *do not* always wait for a tape to be called up for use by the thalamocortical system, the self (see, for example, Persinger and Makarec 1992). In fact, the activity in the basal ganglia is running all the time, playing motor patterns and snippets of motor patterns amongst and between themselves—and because of the odd, re-entrant inhibitory connectivity amongst and between these nuclei, they seem to act as a continuous, random, motor pattern noise generator. Here and there, a pattern or portion of a pattern escapes, without its apparent emotional counterpart, into the context of the thalamocortical system—and suddenly you hear a song in your head or out of seemingly nowhere find yourself anxious to play tennis. Things sometimes just come to us. For some, the things that come are truly unique; Mozart said *his music came to him,* uninterrupted.

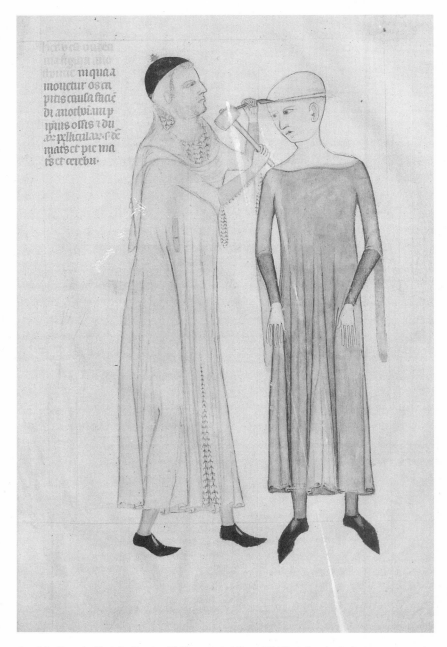

Art Medieval, *Gui de Pavie,* "*Liber notiablium Phillipi Septimi, francorum regis, a libris Galieni extractus.*" *Médicin découpant la boite cranienne d'un malade,* Italy, 1345. Miniature. Chantilly, Musée Conde. Lauros-Giraudon.

9

Of Learning and Memory

Biology's Need to Learn and Remember

Although fixed action patterns (FAPs) constitute an extremely useful set of tools that the nervous system has evolved, we know that by their very nature they are also quite limited; there are boundaries to what a given FAP can do. Given the changing world that all actively moving organisms live in, FAPs must therefore be capable of being modified in their range and thus in their circuitry. Suppose that all FAPs were as rigidly wired in their function (and range of functions) as is the scratch reflex that we saw in chapter 7. The wonders of such an event as human language and its necessary adaptability to the complexity of human communication and thought simply would not have happened. The automatic motor patterns that FAPs truly are must remember and become adaptable to these changes for survival. In an ontogenetic sense they do so by embedding the changes in the body and its parts as a child grows; the nervous system modifies to match the change (see Edelman 1993; Singer 1995). This flexibility is seen as well in the phylogenetic sense, in that such adaptability must be available and the results capable of internalization—not, of course, that we will inherit our parents' specific motor memories, in a Lamarckian sense.

In the ontogenetic sense, a tightrope walker must learn to modify particular FAPs that relate to balance and the reflexes of balance compensation. For the right foot/left foot spinally generated FAP of walking— walking on a line in the sidewalk and walking on a tightrope or wire are not much different at all: simply ask the step cycle to follow a straight line. The sensory feedback, however, is drastically different between the two. There is much more need for compensatory balance adjustment in the case of tightrope walking because the area for foot placement is so limited and because the rope moves in response to the body's movements, whereas a line in the sidewalk does not. The major difference, however, is a contextual one, and a serious one at that. With tightrope walking, if you lose your balance, you may die. Under such circumstances, "easy does it" is the watchword: the goal is to have the rope move as little as possible. This is an example of on-line modification (remember that a FAP can only be modified once it has been activated) of a relatively hard wired FAP (all balance reflexes are fairly hard wired, being very old). It is not at all dissimilar to the modification we employed in saving Mother's Etruscan vase, with the exception that here, the wrong move could be fatal.

Repetition

There is another difference in the modification of these two FAPs that highlights an important aspect of learning and memory that we will discuss throughout this chapter: the issue of repetition. Extremely contained and controlled balance reflexes are honed with practice by tightrope walkers, just as the incredible finger dexterity of a violin player is honed slowly over time, with practice and repetition. This is an on-line modification, but these efforts to modify also add up over time, through repetition. Later we will look at the neuronal mechanisms that listen to and make note of frequently occurring patterns of activity, and how these neuronal mechanisms may alter the level of translated significance that a given pattern of activity has within the internal context. If a particular pattern of activity means "shadow," which usually means "predator," which then usually means "run away," intrinsic properties of the associated neurons may streamline this circuit so that the composite significance of these associations is elevated and hastened: shadow now means immediately release the FAP of "run." A change in internal significance may also be understood in other ways. I see a person for the first time, and his face is represented by a particular pattern of activity of certain, specified neurons. Over the years, this individual becomes my best friend. The internal significance of the pattern of activity that represents this person's face has changed quite a bit from the first time I saw him, even though the pattern of activity representing his face has not changed much at all.

Repetition and practice are not the only route by which the nervous system becomes modified or learns. It is possible to embed properties and events of the body, indeed properties and events of the external world— in a *single* trial fashion. As the reader might guess, this form of learning has everything to do with the prevailing internal context at the time, the particular emotional status. This is an extremely important aspect of learning and we shall discuss this more deeply later in the chapter.

Not unexpectedly, learning, remembering, and adapting FAPs can be seen at the phylogenetic level as well. For instance, over the millennia, in certain species, the FAP of swimming became modified to that of crawling. In many species, the FAPs of breathing and swallowing slowly became modified in their functional range to work together, producing the extremely important FAP known as vocalization. When we ponder the concepts of learning and memory, however, what seem most often to come to mind are the wonders of human capability. The immense amount of knowledge some people acquire from years of education, or the ability to recall a singular event from one's childhood decades later, as clearly as if one were living it again, is what generally comes to mind when thinking of human memory. But one should keep in mind that the neuronal mechanisms subserving these fantastic capacities came to us, as do all things physiological, by the long evolutionary processes of trial and error. For our nervous systems—for *us*—to be able to learn and remember means that evolution not only had to learn and remember, but that it had to learn and remember *how* to learn and remember. *That we* may learn is the unplanned but rather thoroughly born out product of natural selection. *What* we or any creature may learn, however, is a product of the myriad needs and events experienced during development, a rich dream called our personal lives that vanishes leaving no immediate biological legacy. Our memories die with us.

Jumping to Conclusions Over the Millennia: Biological Being and Becoming

At this period in neuroscience, the issues of learning and memory are central. Indeed, the ability to learn is viewed as critical for bettering ourselves within the practical world in which we live. And although this arguably may be true, to some within the field of neuroscience memory itself *is* the basis for the functioning of the nervous system. This *tabula rasa* perspective posits that although the brain is fully wired at birth, ripe with the potential to learn, it has not learned *anything* yet. In fact, it still needs to learn *everything,* a feat that presumably occurs during those vague, shimmering days of infancy. A good example of this posture is the view that speech is fundamentally developed purely from reinforcement and feedback (Skinner 1986). The brain is thus viewed as a "learning machine," a machine that, from its blank slate beginning, simply acquires and accrues experience as memory files upon memory files. This view contrasts with another that I feel reflects a more accurate and circumspect grasping of brain function, one that recognizes the ability of the nervous system to modify itself on the basis of experience. It also recognizes that we basically learn what, at some level, we already know (see, for example, Hadders-Algra et al. 1997, on the development of postural control in infants, and Jusczyk and Bertoncini 1988; Locke 1990; Wexler 1990, on the development of language).

In other words, we are born with a well-wired brain and an incredible amount of knowledge derived from the genetic wiring of our brains. This is easily demonstrated by the existence of such professions as neurology or psychiatry, which *de facto* expect that brain damage in one person will produce similar symptoms in all patients with a similar lesion. In other words, people never learn so much that their neurology becomes fundamentally different from that of a completely uneducated person.

WHAT ABOUT NEUROPLASTICITY?

Phylogenetic Memory: "Basic Connectivity"

It was evolution's task to learn and slowly fine tune the appropriate forms, the structural morphologies that added to the survivability of a given species. By so doing, it brought together the world of our external bodies with our brains. The result was the opposable thumb, the tail of a rat, the nose of a kitten, even the shape of the brain. This kind of memory would be considered phylogenetic; these structural forms are present at birth and do not have to be learned during development, within the short period known as a single lifetime. Such structural memory determines species form, the whole animal, and organ *architectures* that we see echoed across the millennia (figure 9.1).

But the phylogenetic memory of structural form that expresses itself at birth is not enough. Although the dancing eyes of a newborn child may be beguiling, if these eyes do not function, one is justified in asking what the purpose is of the phylogenetic memory of form. Another type of memory must be resident in a creature at birth: that which uniquely marries form with *function*. A muscle cell is nothing if it cannot contract (unless one is an electric fish in which some muscles have been modified to become electricity generating organs; Bennett and Pappas 1983). A neuron, with its beautiful and intricate dendritic and axonal branchings,

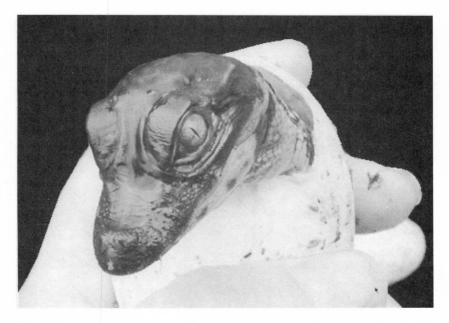

Figure 9.1
Photograph of a caiman hatchling, exhibiting many of the same capabilities at birth as its fully grown parent.

is nothing if it does not communicate with other neurons or a muscle or a gland (unless one is another type of electric fish in which the nerve terminal themselves became another type of electricity generating organ; Bennett et al. 1989).

Dynamic Memory: "Circuit in Action"

We see intertwined into the organ architecture (the plant) a second type of memory, as phylogenetically old as that providing structure, the *electrochemical dynamic structures* (the basic intrinsic activity of the brain prior to experience) that inhabit our brains and that define "us." Neuronal connectivity and the electrochemical "music" it supports is the evolutionary memory that allows the intrinsic oscillatory properties of excitable cells to be present and to represent external reality in a different geometry. These properties allow precise impedance matching that supports electrochemical neuronal communication, the critical functional glue and the basic coinage that assembles together specific functional modules present at birth and resident from generation to generation.

Combined, these two types of memory provide the structural and functional *a prioris* of the body and brain. These are, for example, that we have legs and that these legs work, and that neurons weave themselves during development into the specific functional modules that we call the lobes, fiber bundles, and nuclei of the brain. Regardless of what we may do in our lifetimes, we cannot unlearn the vastly intricate circuitry of the occipital lobe, or what we call visual cortex, the central area that processes the perception of vision unless, of course, our eyes fail us totally when we are very young. We may come to learn the word that humans agree denotes "green," but that we *perceive* "green-ness" is not learned ontogenetically; it has been learned and remembered phylogenetically. This perception is hardwired, and barring damage to the CNS, is an ability we can neither learn nor unlearn—it is no longer within our biological capabilities to do so.

Working in tandem, structural and electrical memory thus provide for the body and brain at birth a beautiful biological state of being and becoming—being, in the sense that functional structures, hands, mouths,

FAPs, and the like are present at birth; becoming, in that the whole system may adapt to the scaling changes imposed on our bodies as we grow during development, or deconstruct with aging. The nervous system and its machinations must be able to innervate and adapt to any type of body. The nervous system during development does not know how tall you will be or how wide apart your eyes will end up being: it must adapt functionally to a body it has never "seen" before. And yet, at all stages of development, the nervous system adapts so that the functioning of any module is unimpaired as it is scaled through the changes in the body's size and relative proportions. Your feet are growing, but your legs grow faster. What does this do to the efficiency of the FAP of walking? Not much!

The functional geometry of the nervous system discussed in chapter 3 must adapt to the functional geometry of an unseen body, and must do so continuously as this functional geometry of the body changes during development. This functional adaptation is necessarily activity-dependent; at all times the dialogue between the neurons and their target muscles (or organs) during ontogeny is actively driven and the embedding process has everything to do with the repetition of activity patterns that we spoke of earlier.

The Prewireness of Brain Function

Let us compare this phylogenetic memory with the *tabula rasa* viewpoint that the nervous system learns how to learn after birth, during development, and that no learning could have occurred prior to birth. Consider for a moment the well known wild life film clip where we see a herd of wildebeests milling around contentedly on a hot African veldt. We see a very pregnant female moments away from birth. The camera drifts to the periphery and shows three or four lions approaching the herd, clearly on the hunt. The pregnant female, frozen to where she stands, is in midbirth, and one lion, still a long way away, spots her. Within five seconds of the calf's birth, the lion strikes. The mother protects, warding off the first attempt. The terrified calf, still in the process of righting itself on wet, wobbly, and spindly legs, awkwardly begins to run away from the lion, darting frantically and successfully evading the attacker, but not for long.

The lion quickly closes the distance and with a single, teeth-bared lunge brings the calf down by its throat; within seconds the calf's short life is over.

This little film clip of the brutal realities of life in the wild highlights a few specific and salient points. First of all, we see that the FAP of running (walking, gait, etc.) is very much in place, prewired and functional, at birth. It is possible, from the *tabula rasa* point of view, to argue that those five seconds between birth and actual running were enough to allow ontogeny to teach the newborn calf how to run, but this is not only unconvincing from an intuitive standpoint, but from a physiological one as well. Even a single working synapse would have problems stabilizing this quickly. Second, the *tabula rasa* perspective argues that learning only occurs in the face of sensory experience. In that case, our newborn calf would have had to learn *how* to run through trial and error. But it ran, granted not as well as an adult, and it did so at its first need to do so. The trial and error of learning how to run must have occurred over phylogeny. This ability and the ability to modify the underlying FAP once it is set into action (the ability to dart this way then that) was evidently instilled as a functional module at birth. Running is simply too critical to survival for this animal to have to learn and embed its functionality *de novo* during ontogeny, generation after generation. Phylogeny has put this FAP into place in the same way as the calf begins breathing regularly at birth.

A second aspect of the film brings to light another serious difference with the *tabula rasa* perspective of learning and memory. In chapter 8 we came to understand that motor FAPs are only released into action by appropriately associated emotional states (though not always "appropriate," as we saw in the case of Tourette's Syndrome). In the case of the newborn calf, the emotional state was that of fear, and thus fear drove the release of the FAP of running. What does this tell us? It tells us that particular emotional states, as is the case for FAPs, are also prewired and operative at birth. Within five seconds of being born, this calf is capable of taking in the specific content of his external world (a lion is coming). He contextually sizes up this content (lion means danger), he implements an appropriate emotional state (danger means fear), and then acts on this internal contextual construct, this sensorimotor image that says fear means "run!" But it doesn't only mean "run," it means attempt to evade the attacker by dodging, i.e., abruptly changing the direction of flight. This sequence indicates that the internal functional matrix we spoke of in chapter 3, the internal functional space that tensorially relates the content of the external world with the ongoing context of the internal world, is itself prewired and ready to do what it does at birth. This also means that *the capacity to have consciousness is a phylogenetic, functional a priori.*

A Third Type of Memory: "Learning from Experience," Practice, Practice, and More Practice

So what can one say about *memory and learning*? Let's formally introduce a third type of memory, one we have already spoken of at length indirectly: that of "referential memory," the type of memory we most commonly think of when we think of the term "memory." Let's be clear: this third type is based on the other two (i.e., body architecture and basic functional brain wiring) and functions by subtly modifying the structural and dynamic properties of brain connectivity, but it is also fundamentally different. It embeds the external world and its properties. This is the functional capability of the brain that allows us to remember the *particular* world each one of us lives in, as opposed to the "all possible worlds" prewired at birth. In other words, the first two types of memory combined provide for the third type, embedding our body properties into the neuronal networkings (internal functional space) of our brains and the expected projections of this internal reference to the external world. Indeed, this third type of memory allows embedding the properties of the *external* world into this internal functional matrix that is generated by the first two types of memory (figure 9.2).

Where the first two types represent the memory accrued and pruned over many lifetimes, as an organism's qualities and characteristics that have been naturally selected for, the referential memory represents that which has accrued during development and throughout a single lifetime. It is an intrinsic capability that aids the predictive properties of the brain and thus contributes fundamentally to an organism's survival. These differing constructs must resonate for a singular, predictive sensorimotor image to be useful: "move toward light if you are selecting a key from

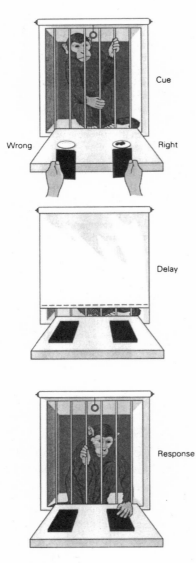

Cue

Wrong   Right

Delay

Response

Figure 9.2
Working memory. A delayed response task tests the functioning of the prefrontal cortex in the functioning of working memory. A monkey briefly views a target stimulus, which in this case is a morsel of food. After some delay, the animal is allowed to retrieve the food. The experimenter randomly varies the location of the food between trials, so that each response tests only the animal's short-term retention of visual and spatial information. The relevant information is not present at the time the response is elicited. Behavior is guided by the internal representation of the rewarded location. (From Goldman-Rakic 1992, p. 112.)

your key-chain." It is the ability to hold the detail of significant content of the external world within the momentary internal context generated by the thalamocortical system. It is also the ability to bring constructs of significance from their moorings in memory should the predictive demands of the prevailing internal context need to do so. Something may be committed to memory and then it may be retrieved or remembered. "Lions typically go there, and so I will remember not to go there if I don't absolutely have to." And so the whole social ecology of, let's say, a watering hole, is based on such memories by the participants, with well-defined access times and a well-defined social order.

And so it is that this third type of referential memory embeds, into the functional matrix generated by the first two types of memory, the properties of the particular world within which a given organism survives. This is so because the system, as we saw in chapter 3, makes attractors based on repetition. If the system has "seen" something before (a particular pattern of electrical activity), it will recognize this pattern better and better each time it is presented; the system will then also coactivate familiar, associated patterns of already embedded patterns of activity. Moreover, the pattern of ensemble firing in a given sensory cortex eventually associates and resonates with neurons in the cortical area that deal with related subjects (visual thalamocortical sites with face recognition thalamocortical sites, for example). Such and such a construct pattern gains significance as it comes to mean, say, the face that is my grandson's. Through repetition and simultaneity, this conglomerate activity pattern becomes associated with particular activity in the language-generating areas of the brain and soon it will be impossible not to have the association of my grandson's face with the internal "hearing" of his name. Quite similarly, a particular snippet of a song is randomly released from the basal ganglia; this fragment of a FAP then brings with it the internal visual of when you heard this song last or perhaps where you were and what you were doing when you first heard it.

This third type of memory can be exemplified very easily. A friend I had not seen for a while came to stay in my house for a few days. After he left, the images I recalled were of his face and some of the conversations that we had. It seems apparent that this type of recall will be more vivid immediately after a conversation, as it is a form of working memory (see below; Goldman-Rakic 1987) or current event memory, no different from that used in remembering where you left the book you recently purchased. This memory may vanish in a few days, leaving, strangely enough, the nagging feeling that you can remember where you left it. If, on the other hand, your friend accidentally sets fire to your house, you will remember his visit for the rest of your life. This is known as a memorable occasion, and one that is clearly referential. It becomes transferred into long-term memory as "things we will never forget." And so, referential memory can be short term (kept for a short time, "where in the parking lot is my car?") as opposed to long term, the friend who burned my house down.

Implicit and Explicit Memory

Referential memory of the long term variety can be subdivided further into implicit and explicit types (Milner et al. 1998). Anyone who has attempted to learn to play a musical instrument knows that "practice makes perfect." The old story of the tourist asking the New Yorker, "How do you get to Carnegie Hall?" and being told "Practice" tells it all. During a single lifetime, we have seen with the likes of a Jascha Heifetz that such perfection rests largely with the nurture aspect of the nature/ nurture equation; however, it also depends on the natural talents of the individual. That is something many have learned the hard way.

Explicit memory, also known as declarative or conscious memory, generally refers to the memory underlying the conscious recollection of things, such as faces, names of objects, past experiences. It has also been further subdivided into two possibly distinct aspects of the retrieval process (Schacter 1987): the voluntary, intentional retrieval of a memory, and the subjective, conscious awareness of having remembered it (Tulving 1983). Implicit memory, nondeclarative or nonconscious memory, is the unconscious, unintentional retrieval of memory for performance of a learned activity or skill. One carries out such a task unaware of that which one has learned and "retrieved" from memory (for recent reviews of explicit and implicit memory, see, for example: Estevez-Gonzalez et al. 1997; Verfaellie and Keane 1997; Milner et al. 1998; Schacter and Buckner 1998; Schachter et al. 1998; Wagner and Gabrieli

1998; see also Rovee-Collier 1997, on memory studies in infants, for an interesting challenge to the limiting definition of explicit memory as confined exclusively to "conscious" recollection).

For Jascha Heifitz, knowing how to draw the bow across the string to produce an exquisite tone is an example of this implicit memory. It is a highly refined, learned motor skill in which the memory of that learning is applied with each stroke of the bow, but to which the artist has no conscious access at that moment.

That these two types of memory are functionally separate and separable from one another in more than a semantical sense emerged from studies begun in the 1950s with amnesic patients who had in most cases undergone medial temporal lobectomy for intractable epilepsy. These patients had suffered a loss of the ability to acquire new memories of places, names, events, or people. Although they could hold an image in their minds for a short time, as soon as attention was diverted that image was irretrievably lost, until re-experienced as something entirely novel and unfamiliar. Most famous among these was "HM," studied extensively over many years (Scoville 1954; Scoville and Milner 1957; Penfield and Milner 1958).

Surprising to the investigators at that time, such patients could be taught motor skills that they retained quite well, usually along a normal learning curve, yet having no conscious recollection of ever having done the task before (Milner 1962) (see figure 9.2). Thus the patient with obliterated explicit memory for recently acquired information had intact motor skill learning, the first type of implicit memory clearly distinguishable as mediated by neural substrates different from those of "remembering." At the end of 30 trials spread over three days, the patient HM was able to attain and retain a fairly difficult drawing skill (figure 9.3), yet when presented with the task after the three-day learning period he had no idea that he had ever done the task before. It was "unfamiliar" to him.

A more curious and astounding form of implicit memory is revealed with amnesic patients asked to identify line drawings of common objects made "sketchy" and difficult to identify by removing many of the contours of the object. After successive presentations, patients became more adept at perceiving and identifying what they were shown, and this

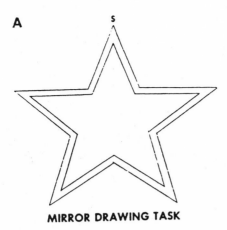

MIRROR DRAWING TASK

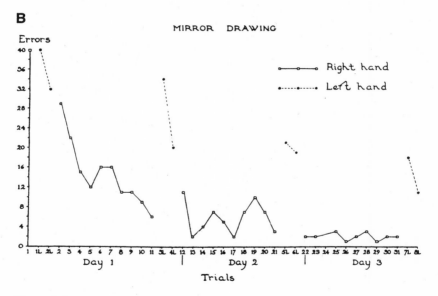

Figure 9.3
(*A*) Improvement in a task that involved the learning of skilled movements. In this test, the patient HM was taught to trace a line between the two outlines of a star, beginning at point S, while viewing his hand and the star in a mirror. His drawing improved steadily over the three days of testing, even though at each ensuing session he had no idea that he had ever done the task before. The graph in (*B*) plots the number of times during each trial that HM strayed outside the boundaries as he drew the star. (From Milner et al. 1998, figure 2, p. 449; after Milner 1962).

ability was retained over many weeks of testing. But again, when presented with the tasks, patients did not remember ever performing the test before. This "perceptual learning," as it was called by Brenda Milner, is what we now refer to as priming (Milner et al. 1968; Warrington and Weiskrantz 1968; see Milner et al. 1998).

Other types of implicit memory include emotional learning such as fear conditioning (LeDoux 1996, 1998; Davis et al. 1996) and category learning, the ability to learn how to identify and classify objects according to extractable characteristics or features they possess (Weiskrantz 1990; Tulving and Schachter 1990; Reed et al. 1999). From lesion studies in animals and the studies of amnesic patients, and more recently with the advent of neuroimaging including PET (positron emission tomography) and fMRI (functional magnetic resonance imaging), it has been possible to localize the brain regions most closely associated with these types of memory (for review, see Schacter and Buckner 1998). Brain regions that seem to underlie implicit memory include most prominently the amygdala, whereas aspects of explicit memory clearly involve the hippocampus and prefrontal cortex.

So how does this apply to the real world of human behavior? What is the role of explicit versus implicit memory in the learning and then execution of a musical composition in a concert, for example? The previously mastered and memorized composition represents a learned motor skill, and is largely implicit memory. There is simply no time to think about what is the next note you must play. But the process of mastering a new piece, although it represents motor skill learning, nevertheless requires the interplay of explicit and implicit memory. How so? Without intact explicit memory, Jascha Heifitz would not remember from day to day which piece he had chosen to work on previously, or that he had ever worked on that piece before. Nor would he recall what he had accomplished the day before or by analysis of past experience what particular problems in execution should be a focus of today's practice session. In fact, it would not occur to him to have a practice session at all; without close direction from someone else he would be effectively incapable of undertaking the process of learning any new piece, irrespective of his considerable technical skills.

Over 40 years of study have determined that implicit memory underlying the learning of tasks and skills can be completely dissociated from explicit memory, both functionally and anatomically, but the truth is that without explicit memory to guide us virtually all learning would be exclusively "reactive" and primitive. Explicit memory, defined as conscious recollection, the subjective awareness that one is retrieving a memory, provides the crucial context and direction for volitional learning, and by extension all that we "create" external to ourselves. The mutual dependence of these two separate memory processes suggests that they must have evolved together, for the most part, and that they may also share a common developmental timeline as well (see Rovee-Collier 1997; Gerhardstein et al. 2000).

On the Mechanisms for the Acquisition of Memories and for Remembering

Speculations about the neural substrate for learning and memory have abounded for more than a hundred years. At the beginning of this century, Ramon y Cajal, one of the true intellectual and experimental pioneers in neuroscience, introduced the so-called neuron doctrine, that all brains are the wiring product of individual cells, the neurons. He also proposed that long-term learning occurs by strengthening synaptic connections (chapter 4) and through the generation of new connections among neurons (Ramón y Cajal 1911).

As mentioned above, in recent times investigators have proposed that short-term or "working" memory is supported by ongoing activity that re-enters a neuronal loop (Goldman-Rakic et al. 1990; Goldman-Rakic 1996; Paulesu et al. 1993). This is a bit like continuously repeating a phone number to oneself in order to remember it while dialing the phone, a somewhat risky substitute for writing the number down. This may be supported by ongoing electrical activity produced by synaptic feedback, or by the persistent activation of neurons by their intrinsic properties (Camperi and Wang 1998). Good examples have been proposed for working memory (Chelazzi et al. 1998; Glassman 1999) and for the maintenance of eye position during gaze (Hayhoe et al. 1998; McPeek et al. 1999). Since the time of Donald O. Hebb (1953); associative memory has been equated with long-term potentiation (LTP) and long-term depression (LTD) (see Goldman-Rakic et al. 1990, and Goldman-Rakic 1996, for reviews). These mechanisms are described by the ability that synapses have to modify the amount of transmitter released by a

A Experimental setup

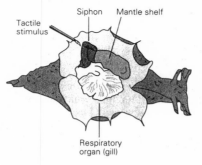

B Gill-withdrawal reflex circuit

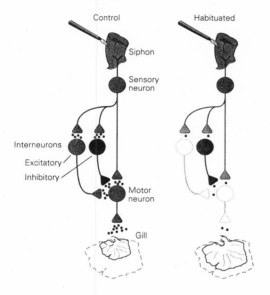

Figure 9.4
The cellular mechanisms of habituation, as illustrated with the gill-withdrawal reflex of the marine snail, *Aplysia*. (*A*) A dorsal view of *Aplysia* illustrates the respiratory organ (gill), which is normally covered by the mantle shelf. The mantle shelf ends in the siphon, a fleshy spout used to expel seawater and waste. A tactile stimulus to the siphon elicits the gill-withdrawal reflex. Repeated stimuli lead to habituation. (*B*) This simplified circuit shows key elements involved in the gill-withdrawal reflex as well as sites involved in habituation. In this circuit about 24 mechanoreceptors in the abdominal ganglion innervate the gill and with several groups of excitatory and inhibitory interneurons that synapse on the motor neurons. (Only one of each type of neuron is shown here.) Repeated stimulation of the siphon leads to a depression of synaptic transmission between the sensory and motor neurons as well as between certain interneurons and the motor cells. (From Kandel et al. 2000, figure 63-1, p. 1248).

presynaptic action potential, or the ability that the postsynaptic cell has to produce postsynaptic receptors that make the receiving cell more (LTP) or less (LTD) sensitive. Indeed, much of the detail concerning how such synaptic modifications are implemented was first demonstrated in invertebrates (for a review, see Kandel et al. 2000). Moreover, many of the molecular steps involved in such modifications are beginning to be understood in detail (Kandel et al. 2000).

Regardless of the sweat and toil we may put in during our lives, the details of the electrical current flow through neuronal membranes that comprises our learning (or the memory of what we have learned) is something we cannot pass on to our offspring. We cannot pass it on in the way that we may pass on the family genes that give that signature nose, the color of eyes, or the predisposition to corpulence. Why is it that what is learned during ontogeny does not find its way through the familial conduit of DNA to the next generation? Why indeed, particularly if repetition seems to have so solidly engrained something, such as our native language, our sense of self, something we are with *every day* of our lives?

Phylogenetic and Referential Memory

The explanation for why we cannot pass on our memories lies in our fathoming of time and our definition of significance, phylogenetic versus referential. What we deem significant, which can only be determined from the perspective of the seat of prediction, the self, and what the self has experienced and juxtaposed over a single lifetime, are not what natural selection considers noteworthy or preservable. What do we hold, in our lifetimes, as significant? We run through the memories—graduation, a particular Christmas morning, the birth of a child—as if they are filed nicely in some sort of an emotional Rolodex, and certain events from our childhood may stick with us all our lives.

But although these events clearly highlight our lives, indeed *are* our lives, they mean very little to biological evolution, for they are too variable, too case-specific at the individual level, and have little or no impact on the species as a whole. Moreover, they are not repetitive, consistent, or frequent enough in the time frames that phylogeny, natural selection, requires for incorporation into the genomic blueprint. As short-term memory is to individuals, so is long-term memory in individuals just short term to the species. The difference lies in that the long-term memory of individuals can only be kept in place by social culture. Genetic memory (long term in species terms) is present at birth, *as memory that occurs in the absence of sensory experience.* Such memories were written directly into our genetic code by the myriad of small mutations occurring in our genome over time and brought to light by natural selection. Beneficial adaptations that become genomic are not so because of practice. Our teeth are inherited, and even though we may take care to conscientiously eat only harder foods throughout life to make our teeth stronger and more capable, this effort will have no impact on the teeth that our children inherit. That's about it for one lifetime, unless, over the millennia, you've proven a case for stronger teeth increasing productive fitness—in other words, if there was a positive selection for those random event mutations that aided one's ability to consume foods facilitating survival for the successful reproduction of viable offspring. Thus we have our teeth, thus their shape (see, for example, Brown 1983; Krishtalka et al. 1990; Plavcan 1993; Stock et al. 1997).

We see the same difference between phylogenetic and ontogenetic memory if we look at human language. Clearly, any form of intraspecies communication aids in survival, and there is no exception in the case of humans. How and from where human language developed will be handled in detail in chapter 10. For our purposes here, suffice it to say that the fact *that* we can have language is a property of the nervous system present at birth, a phylogenetic *a priori*. During ontogeny, the perception of phonemes a child has at birth is very quickly reduced to the perception of only those phonemes used in his/her native language. We may not properly recognize the sounds specific to those languages we are not exposed to during our childhood (Kuhl et al. 1997). The acquisition of our native language is implemented via linguistically prespecified rules (Chomsky 1980) through a process of selective use and repetition (Jusczyk and Bertoncini 1988; Locke 1990; Wexler 1990; Greenfield and Savage-Rumbaugh 1993; Werker and Tees 1999), but it is not through the process of practice and repetition that this language ability is with us, but rather only the particular way we use it. If phylogenetic memory were Lamarckian, children in France would be born predisposed to speak French, and there is no such genetic predisposition to human language. "Culture" is simply not old enough or consistent enough for natural selection to pay attention to it.

Knowledge in the Absence of Experience

As far as the brain and body are concerned, we must work with what we have, and what we are. For the most part, this very specific connectivity is acquired in the *absence* of experience. This means that during ontogeny, functionally capable and correct brain circuits are generated in the total absence of sensory input. For example, in the mammalian visual system, the eye itself and all of the functional connectivity ultimately capable of supporting vision is built *completely* in the absence of light input; this intrinsic connectivity is formed while the animal is still in the womb. Many years ago, David Hubel and Torsten Wiesel described how neurons in the visual cortex of a newborn monkey respond selectively to lines of particular orientation and movement direction even though the animal had never seen lines before (Hubel and Wiesel 1963, 1974, 1977; Wiesel and Hubel 1974; Hubel et al. 1976). In this case it is not reasonable to say that the brain "learned," but rather that the neuronal connectivity of the brain must have been specified and driven by factors other than (experiential) learning. These factors most likely derived from the intrinsic electrical properties of the relevant cells (recall motricity climbing up the neuraxis in chapters 2 and 3), timed associated neural growth factors, interactions among developing and migrating axonal fibers, and the respective neurons receiving the terminals of these migrating fibers. These receiving cells may then accept or deny access to their receptors by allowing or denying certain cell-to-cell adhesion events. Very importantly, all of these events are an ontogenetic prelude to sensory input-evoked synaptic transmission.

This scenario is a clear strike against the *tabula rasa* concept of brain function, which argues that the neural connectivity that supports specific given functions is driven by sensory experience. It is not possible for sensory derived experience in the brain or its neuronal circuits to occur in the absence of sensory evoked synaptic transmission. This must be distinguished from the spontaneous electrical activity that is present in our sense organs in the absence of sensory input, as happens for instance in the eye, where retinal neurons fire spontaneously prior to birth. This activity, which is required for the establishment of normal wiring in the visual system (Penn et al. 1998; Cook et al. 1999; Eglen 1999), is not driven by the presence or absence of specific external stimuli.

What Changes When We Learn

During our lifetimes, what we add to these preordained patterns are the modifications that underlie learning and memory, the new connections, the changes at the protein level that influence specific synaptic efficiency. Measurable modifications and additions such as changes in muscle tone and density from exercise and use are minimal, however, when compared to what we *do* behaviorally with those modifications. Variation in both neuronal architecture and composition at the molecular level of cells that make up the cortical language areas of a person who speaks only French *versus* one who speaks only Spanish may be so small that one could not detect any differences. Yet each of these languages represents entirely different worlds to a person trained in the other. Notwithstanding the recent evidence of ongoing neurogenesis (generation of new neurons) in the mature primate brain (Gould et al. 1999), ontogenetically speaking, learning and memory constitute only very slight modifications of elements or modules within the functional architecture already determined by phylogeny, already present at birth.

And so, if one were asked to what extent the brain is prewired by nature and to what extent it is modified by the nurturing provided by experience and by learning, my view would have to be that the system is, for the most part, genetically determined. There are powerful arguments for this line of thinking, supported by the aforementioned work of Hubel and Wiesel in vision, Mountcastle in somatosensory systems (Mountcastle 1979, 1997, 1998), and Chomsky in language (Chomsky 1959, 1964, 1986).

The basic brain circuitry for these functions is not acquired through learning. If central connectivity were seriously modified during development by learning, neurology as such would be impossible. This is so because the normative functioning of the brain would ultimately modify the structure of the individual's brain to such a great extent that it would be impossible to know where the visual cortex is or the particular function of any part of the brain from one person to another. Moreover, consider that our eyes are for the most part not perfectly aligned because the two sides of our heads are not precisely symmetrical and that the morphology of the eyes and their associated muscles may not be precisely the same. Thus, when the eyes are relaxed they may well not be parfocal (see

Braddick 1996 for discussion of binocularity development in infants). And yet when we look at something, our eyes generally align quite beautifully, and realign when we look at an object that is near to us as opposed to one that is far away (see Miles 1999, for discussion of visual stabilization mechanisms). We also know that certain substances that alter the function of the nervous system, such as alcohol, may generate double vision when taken in sufficient quantities (Miller 1992). This double vision (diplopia) occurs because the eyes are no longer perfectly aligned.

The nervous system is clearly capable of correcting for such deviations, but only up to a point. For reasons of peripheral trauma or congenital central miswiring, a person may demonstrate a squint (strabismus). The nervous system may not be capable of correcting for it if the deviation is too large, as evidenced by the many children who effectively lack depth perception (stereopsis) due to congenital strabismus (Archer et al. 1986; Weinstock et al. 1998). This means then that the inherent ability to learn or the ability to correct errors has a rather clear range. The system might be able to modify this range *slightly* but always at a cost of some other function being lost. It is very similar to athletes, where by necessity, advanced specialization in one sport ultimately results in the loss of the ability to become competitive in another type of sport at the same advanced level. For the same reasons there are very few virtuosi in more than one instrument and none that are virtuoso in *all* instruments.

Here again, perhaps the best example that we know of is the acquisition of language, in particular, the acquisition of the phonemes that characterize a certain language (See Winkler et al. 1999). Unless these are learned within a particular period of time, the possibility of acquisition or retention of these specific phonemes will be irreversibly lost (Kuhl et al. 1997; Kuhl 2000). The bottom line then, is that one can learn a particular language, but only at the expense of the ability to learn other languages to the same extent (Logan et al. 1991). This is a particularly contentious issue, as many people may consider themselves articulate, to the point of eloquence, in more than one language. Generally, upon close scrutiny, that is rarely, if ever, the case. Similarly, consider that language can be understood and executed at only certain speeds. That is to say, if the rate at which words are spoken were increased as little as ten-fold, we would never be able to understand the speech or execute it as such (Llinás et al. 1998). This means that within the realm of the possible, not only is language very much already preset, but the boundaries of language, outside of which one can no longer learn or adapt to it, are also preset. From this point of view, we are really quite limited to what we already know (are phylogenetically prewired to express) and the range of adaptability of a particular function. Such limits of adaptability apply to *everything* we do or learn.

The Requirements for Learning Given by Nature

We may feel a touch slighted by the fact that the self is fundamentally just a convenient construct on the part of the nervous system to centralize and thus coordinate its predictive properties. We, our egos, also may feel a little deflated by the fact that learning, and subsequently what goes into memory, comes only from the honing of properties that are already present in our nervous systems at birth.

Furthermore, this honing operation, which we can measure as changes in the number of synaptic contacts within a given circuit, as well as the efficiency of given synaptic contacts, is very, very small when we compare such measured events to what functionally comes from them. These are the languages we learn, the people and places we have committed to memory, and the specific education we attained long ago and continue to utilize every day. Yet although our inferior olivary nuclei and visual pathways look alike, our visual memories are totally different. One would expect that in the face of all these sensorimotor images available to us, more serious physiological modifications would have occurred within the nervous system, but the actual synaptic modifications that produce these memories are very slight. The range limits of learning, in the physiological sense, help define and dictate our commonality. If there were not preset physiological limits within which the speed of perceivable language production is constrained, the very thread of commonality providing for human to human language development may never have been selected for. Phylogeny determines that green is pretty much green to all our visual systems. These limitations to learning and memory are as valuable in our consensus dealings with the external world as is the ability to learn.

We learn to facilitate nervous system function in order to adapt to the requirements given by nature, by the world in which we live. Although the details of the external world seem to be of the ontogenetic realm, the on-line, "what's happening right now" realm, the significance of such detail may be given by the phylogenetically preset characteristics of the organism. For example, if an animal does not digest grass and wants to survive, it may have to learn to hunt other animals. An excellent example of such required learning is the acquisition of hunting skills by carnivorous animals.

The lion who successfully attacked the newborn wildebeest was young once, too. The foundations of the hunting skills this lion employed were innate, but the details, the context-dependent tactics of carnivorous predation, had to be learned.

As cubs, many of the skills of hunting are learned through interaction with littermates during development. Here, through the rough and tumble of play, the cubs learn the parameters of successful pouncing, pawing, and teething, the ins and outs of how to subdue another creature. They also learn the boundaries of these individual skills, when play is no longer play, when biting or pawing hurts and/or frightens.

The above is mainly direct learning, through mostly tactile routes of experience. But the cubs also learn more teleceptively as well, by watching examples shown to them by mother. Mother, or as likely a group of mothers, will take the cubs along on a real hunt, having them watch the action from afar, letting them in closer, perhaps letting the cubs participate if the safety of the situation permits. This is where the cubs learn the very differing tactics of hunting: creeping up and pouncing on a bird is very different from chasing and pulling down a wildebeest. Here is where the cub learns indirectly about the way another animal's brain works: about the typical running patterns of a gazelle; that a wild boar will likely turn and launch its own attack; about the body posture and attentiveness of a snake that says it will strike *right now*. The cubs are developing their predictive skills, the critical skills needed for survival.

This leads to a very interesting conclusion about the evolution of the nervous system that the reader may well have already realized. We spoke at length in chapter 3 of the need for organisms with nervous systems to move actively within the world in order to embed into their internal functional space the salient properties of the external world. If we look at the development of the cortical mantle across species, we see that the more sophisticated circuitry lies with those creatures that are carnivorous rather than those that graze for their food, the herbivores. This makes perfect phylogenetic and ontogenetic sense: those animals that must seriously compete for their food must have a far greater repertoire of food procuring tactics at their momentary disposal, not to mention that in most cases the food is not obtained without a species-specific stereotypical fight. These animals interact in a far more sophisticated way with their world and this must be reflected in the neural systems underlying these elevated interactions. Again, the ability, the prewired circuitry, is provided phylogenetically and is honed through ontogeny.

Imprinting

Another wonderful example of the properties of learning is that of a widespread phenomenon crucial to survival called "imprinting" (Lorenz 1935, 1937; Tinbergen 1951; Bateson 1966) (figure 9.5), which has also been referred to as "perceptual learning" (Bateson 1966). Imprinting, especially in birds, has been studied in detail. Here we have a situation where particular properties of the external world come to define intrinsic central connectivity so that a particular sound and a particular visual clue in conjunction may be defined to a duckling as meaning, and forever meaning, "mother." That "mother" can be imprinted only once makes intuitive sense; it does not serve a duckling well if it has seven different events in the external world all of which mean mother. A duckling needs its mother and it needs this construct of mother to be its real mother. That only one combination of stimuli comes to mean mother is an intrinsic property of the circuits that embed this maternal representation. An attractor-like property through repetition of a given sequence of stimuli—hear quack, orient to quack, see this big duck—ultimately comes to embed the construct of mother. There is a sensitive period of time during which the repetition of such sequences or combinations of stimuli will come to be embedded. If a duckling is put into isolation directly after birth and kept away from sensory input for a defined period of time, no mother construct will be learned. Even if the actual mother of this duckling is presented after the sensitive period has passed, no mother construct will be embedded: even the real mother will never mean mother (Hess 1972).

The attractor-like properties of the pertinent neuronal circuits are very strong during this critical period for learning—as they must be: a duckling needs to learn mother first and foremost in this world to survive. During the critical period, if the actual mother is taken away, the duckling will imprint as mother such things as a shoe, a bucket, or any object that is repeatedly presented. And so, under these (experimental) conditions, even in the face of its real, urgently quacking mother, the duckling will follow around a shoe pulled by a string, because as far as the duckling knows, this *is* mother, and mother is to be followed.

We may ask why ducklings in the wild don't inadvertently imprint other sequences of stimuli—other things—as mother. Well, it can happen, but the likelihood of the real mother duck being imprinted as mother is

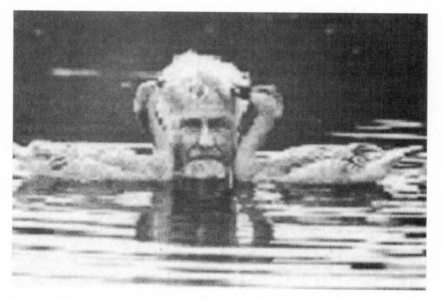

Figure 9.5
Konrad Lorenz out for a swim with geese that were imprinted on him as goslings. See text for more details.

very, very high. Right after birth, the repertoire of sensory events from the external world that a duckling is exposed to is quite narrow (they don't move around much unless mother is nearby). Within that limited amount of sensory exposure, the majority of sensory detail arises from interactions with the actual mother. And so, for the most part, nature does its job and ducklings typically end up with the mothers they are supposed to have.

A very interesting aspect to this is the attractor-like functioning of these circuits that embed the combination of sensory stimuli to mean mother. This is in every way the same as the streamlining of synaptic connectivity mentioned earlier, when shadow meant predator, which meant run away, followed by over-repetition to more beneficially hasten processing to just: "shadow means activate the FAP of running." This is also what we spoke of in chapter 6 concerning the attracting and binding of varied sensory stimuli into a single, unified perceptual construct. Learning the mother construct was no different. The fascinating aspect of all this is that the mother construct, once embedded, can be activated in full by a single sensory component of the complete construct. That is, the mother's quack, when the duckling cannot see the mother, nevertheless means "mother": go to her.

Imprinting is not limited to mother. For example, in the wild, ducks in a brood will imprint to their peers as well as to their mother (Dyer et al. 1989; Dyer and Gottlieb 1990). Imprinting is something that we all do, or rather our nervous systems do. A friend and colleague of mine, a well-known and respected physician, told of a particular incident he experienced during World War II. While serving on a ship in the Navy, there was a particular smell to the paint used throughout the ship. Years and years later, if he smells this particular paint—anywhere, under any conditions—he *hears* the whirring of the ship's engines. It is the attractor aspects of the circuits that have embedded the construct: if your senses allow in one aspect, the system resonates all of the other aspects, (re-)creating the full, internal sensorimotor image or construct. These different sensory related components of a given construct reside in very disparate parts of our cortices and it is neuronal resonance that recombines them for us.

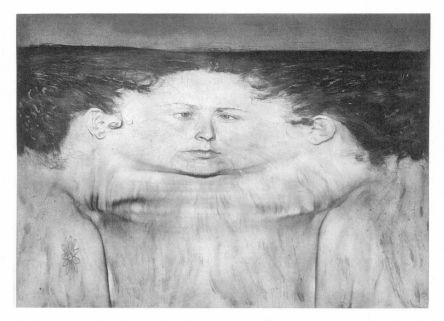

Kiki Smith, *My Blue Lake,* 1994. Photogravure and monoprint, 42-1/2 × 53-1/2″
(108 × 135.9 cm); edition of 41. Photograph by Ellen Page Wilson. Courtesy of
PaceWildenstein.

Qualia from a Neuronal Point of View

KEY CHAPTER

Exorcising the Ghost in the Machine

"Qualia" refers to the quality of entities. The philosopher Willard Quine used the term to denote the feeling character of sensation. I shall use the term qualia to denote subjective experience of *any* type generated by the nervous system (Smart 1959), be it pain (Benini 1998), the color green (Churchland and Churchland, 1998), or the specific timbre of a musical note (see, for general discussions, Gregory 1988, 1989; Leeds 1993; Sommerhoff and MacDorman 1994; Banks 1996; Hubbard 1996; Feinberg 1997). This issue has been discussed at great length from a philosophical point of view (Churchland 1986; Searle 1992, 1998; Dennett 1993; Chalmers 1996, among others).

There are today two similar beliefs concerning the nature of qualia. The first is that qualia represent an epiphenomenon that is not necessary for the acquisition of consciousness (Davis 1982). Second and somewhat related is the belief that while being the basis for consciousness, qualia appeared only in the highest life forms, suggesting that qualia represent a recently evolved central function that is present in only the more advanced brains (Crook 1983). This view relegates the more lowly animals, for example ants, to a realm characterized by the absence of subjective experiences of any kind. It implies that these animals are wired with sets of automatic, reflexively organized circuits that provide for survival by maintaining a successful, albeit purely reactive interaction with the ongoing external world. Although primitive creatures such as ants and cockroaches may be wildly successful, for all practical purposes they are biological automatons.

For those of the elitist camp who believe that qualia are limited to be part of the brain functioning of higher lifeforms, there is another qualia-damning caveat to this view as well: qualia arose accidentally, as an unexpected, perhaps emergent property of the brain's complex circuitry but it is not necessary for properly organized behavior. Those who adhere to this position typically point out that even in the case of qualia-endowed humans the great majority of what goes on in the brain is *not* part of qualia, nor are qualia a part of those events. Rather, they propose that most brain activity has been involved with the more preconscious functions and/or the neuronal goings-on that support motor coordination. Further, they often point out that even these rather infrequently employed aspects of brain function that can *in principle* subserve sensory experience simply may not always do so, particularly if one is momentarily distracted. While watching a tennis match your wallet is stolen— you remember only later that perhaps you did feel something brush your hip or breast pocket. According to these views, qualia are not necessary components or products of brain function, and even if they occasionally are, they are essentially rather fleeting and unreliable.

To me, these views lack a proper evolutionary perspective, which is perhaps why qualia are given so little overall emphasis in the study of brain function. We clearly understand that the functional architecture of the brain is a product of the slow tumblings of evolution and that brain function implements what natural selection has found to be the most beneficial in terms of species survivability. What is not often understood is how deeply related qualia truly are to the evolutionary, functional structure of the brain. My argument is that sensory experience leading to active movement (motricity) through the function of prediction *is* the ultimate reason for the very existence of the central nervous system. If one takes into consideration the fact that perception itself—through *any* sense modality—has become the elaborate process we see now through the course of evolution, then the most parsimonious view is that sensory experience, qualia, *must* be primordial in the global organization of nervous system function. In fact, qualia must represent a significant and influential drive throughout evolution. Allow me to elaborate on this point.

We know from developmental biology that as the nervous system matures, given functions may migrate from one site in the brain to another. A given function may evolve away from a given location during ontogeny and/or over great expanses of evolutionary time. This migration of function can only be accomplished by the migration of the complete neuronal embodiment of that function.

Ontogenetically speaking, the best example of this migration of function is how elasmobranchs oxygenate themselves during embryogenesis (Harris and Whiting 1954). The reader will recall that intrinsic tremor in the musculature itself leads, via electrotonic coupling, to rhythmic, oscillatory movement, thus allowing water flow though the gills and oxygen exchange with the external world and, so vital to life, throughout the egg sack. This form of motricity is "myogenic," for it represents movement born purely from the intrinsic properties of the muscle cells.

How does the migration of function relate to qualia? We have mentioned that over phylogeny the head (rostral) end or pole of an animal has become richer in sense organs, as opposed to their migrating to, say, the foot or the tail. Why? Because of an animal's choice of what will be its "forward" direction of movement. It makes selective sense that sensory organs would migrate to a body location where they are most beneficially utilized, particularly when used in combination.

And so, from the need to sensorially monitor the world within which an animal may move, the head pole becomes richer in sense organs because of the forward movement of the animal. Further, not only do these individual sense organs become richer in their capability of monitoring the external world, the nerve centers associated with and supporting this rostral pole in turn specialize to perform the rapid, predictive decision making that underlies and maintains the holistic behaviors crucial for survival. But more fundamentally, the experience serves to contextualize and to arouse the unity of sensory activation into one global functional state—something akin to "I feel" that acts to mediate decision making. It is clear from this that the head becomes the seat of qualia, having moved from more caudal regions to be supported by and to drive a richer neural connectivity. Understanding this, it seems to me that qualia, sensory experience, must certainly be one of the fundamental neuronal ensemble properties that gave rise to the evolutionary development of the central nervous system. And if qualia play such a crucial role in the phylogenic development of the central nervous system, then it is hard to believe that they play no role, or that the role they play is sketchy or unimportant as many say, in the functioning of our brains during our lifetimes. We shall discuss the importance of qualia—their critical necessity—in the latter parts of this chapter. It is now time, however, to address qualia, what they are, what they must be, from an objective, physiological point of view.

Localizing Qualia

While performing surgery for intractable epilepsy, Wilder Penfield electrically stimulated various aspects of the brains of epileptic patients and asked them to report what sort of sensory experience was elicited by the stimulation. This technique exposes the cerebral cortex with little or no discomfort to the patient, and the patients are fully awake and capable of reporting on what may be occurring to them. What Penfield found (apart from making limbs, fingers, and lips twitch from electrical stimulation of various parts of the motor homunculus) was that very specific sensory experiences could also be elicited by electrical stimulation of somatosensory and associational cortices (Penfield and Rasmussen 1950) (figure 10.1). Such experiences included "hearing" parts of familiar songs or voices and "seeing" a relative or a vista from the past. These were perhaps not as complete as a sensory experience generated by the activation of the sensory pathways themselves, the experiencing of something arising from the external world, or the conscious recollection of a memory, but the simple pulsing of electricity into relatively tiny areas of the cortex gener-

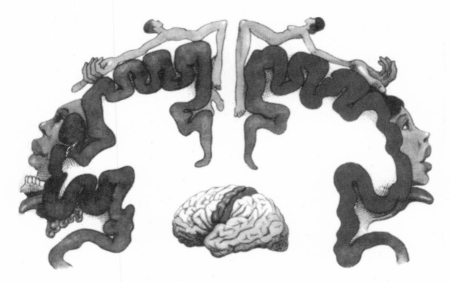

Figure 10.1
Famous maps drawn by Wilder Penfield, showing how each part of the body is represented on two strips of the brain's cerebral cortex, the somatosensory cortex (left), which receives sensations of touch (which he termed the "sensory homunculus"), and the motor cortex (right), which controls movement ("motor homunculus"). On both maps, the fingers, mouth and a few other sensitive areas take up most of the space on both maps. (From Posner and Raichle 1995.)

ated—or recreated—sensory experience in every way similar to the real thing. There is something in a neuronal sense very modular about sensory experience.

In like fashion, we may stimulate, say, the right index finger of our patient with the exposed cortex and look at the very specific neural activity in response to this stimulation in the index finger area of somatosensory cortex.

"What did we stimulate?" the doctor asks.

"My right index finger." The activity of the cells in this part of the cortex would also say yes, the right index finger was indeed stimulated.

Now a very fascinating event may be demonstrated, if we anesthetize either the somatosensory cortex or nuclei of the thalamus related specifically to this pathway of tactile information (as done during a procedure known as a Wada Test to locate the site for the speech center in neurosurgery). When we again stimulate our patient's finger and ask what was stimulated, we inevitably hear: "You didn't stimulate anything yet." We have created with our barbiturate application a complete and immediate disappearance of sensation, of this specific sensory experience, *without any change in connectivity or anatomy of any type.* As this may also be done with local anaesthesia, we must conclude that qualia are indeed fundamentally related to the electrical activity of the brain. All we have done by the application of anesthesia is to modify one single aspect of the function of the nerve cells: the ability to generate particular electrical patterns of activity.

That qualia must be subserved by electrical events at nerve cells makes enormous theoretical sense as well. Think of the unbelievable rapidity with which any sensory stimulus may be analyzed and woven into a stream of consciousness. Bringing to mind the 40-Hz oscillatory activation of the brain and its relation to intrinsic thalamocortical activity, we saw that a quantum of cognition can be measured to be a well defined 12–15 millisecond time epoch. This means that the perceptual capabilities of the central nervous system are such that for two sensory stimuli to be perceived as two distinguishable sensory events, there must be a minimum of 12.5 milliseconds separating these events—otherwise, the brain will register them as a single sensory event (Kristofferson 1984; Llinás and Pare 1991; Llinás and Ribary 1993; Joliet et al. 1994). Such a quantum of cognition requires the patterned activation of millions or even hundreds of millions of cells. Given this, the *only* way that cells would ever be able to generate an event of this coherent nature would be to use electricity as the connecting mode of information flow between them— no other medium we know (that exists within the brain) is even remotely fast enough! If we look at the possible biological events in and about even a single neuron, a 12–15 millisecond time frame of ensemble activity encompassing or employing hundreds of millions of cells poses very serious limitations in terms of the plausible carriers of this type of necessary information flow. Diffusion is far, far too slow and its range of effect is far too short. In these time frames, a given molecule could not get very far from a cell, or very far *into* a cell for that matter, if diffusion were the carrier of ensemble information flow. Electricity is the only medium fast enough and far reaching enough to support the rapid and widespread ensemble activity underlying sensory experience within perceptual time frames envisioned by Charles Sherrington as "the enchanted loom" (1941, p. 225). So we must accept that qualia are triggered by electrical activity in the brain and are made up of events very close in time to the electrical structures that skate over the surfaces of neuronal membranes. These electrical vortices dart this way and that, like sheet lightning that flickers and passes, leaving behind only a faint, short-lasting glow—a sensation to be lit up again as the next sheet of lightning strikes and spreads, forming to us the perception of a continuous web of sensation. Qualia truly are fleeting and discontinuous cellular events for the same physiological reasons that consciousness itself is a fleeting and discontinuous event. That qualia and the self—specifically self-awareness—are related is a topic we shall look into toward the end of the chapter.

Having related qualia to the electrical events of neurons, we can say even more. When considering the large functional events of the central nervous system, such as waking or sleep, not only is electrical activity necessary but electrical activity at particular frequencies, as was discussed in detail in chapter 6 when examining thalamocortical connectivity and function. When we fall into dreamless sleep, non-REM sleep as it is called, we see that this functional state is characterized by slow wave, synchronous delta wave activity (Llinás and Ribary 1993). This whole brain, rhythmic wave pattern is in the .5–4 Hz frequency range and has the largest amplitude of EEG or MEG (magnetoencephalogram) monitored brain activity. Recall from chapter 6 that when in this deep sleep state, sensory input of all types (modalities)is for the most part rejected by the thalamocortical system. Sensory pathways carry their modality-specific information, but this information is not given internal significance; there is in fact no sensory experience whatsoever. Qualia have temporarily ceased to exist!

Similarly, qualia also cease to be during a petit mal seizure where simply, because of the epileptic state, the prominent frequency of brain activity is lowered, without otherwise affecting much or any of the connectivity or the basic, ongoing functioning of the nervous system. All sensory experience—indeed the "person"—is gone. So it is not just electrical activity of neurons that determine qualia, but particular frequency ranges of whole brain activity where qualia may appear and disappear. In simple terms, there are particular types of electrical patterns, global and local, that must be coactivated for feelings to be evoked.

The Functional Geometry of Qualia: Internalized FAPs

What may we say then is the neuronal basis for qualia? To pursue this, I would like to address the subject of qualia from a somewhat theoretical perspective, starting with the motor point of view and based on much of what we have already learned from earlier chapters. Ultimately, motricity is always the product of muscle contraction; we can make no movement through any other means. From this we immediately come to the conclusion that the nervous system works within the context of a final motor effector that is capable of transforming the electrical activity of motor neurons into actual muscular contraction. We may ask by analogy what is the effector, the apparatus for the endpoint expression of *sensory* experience. This is the central question of neuroscience at the present time. The answer is that physiologically we do not know what the effectors of sensory experience are or how they work. We do, however, know the realms of operation of such effectors, that they require electrical, neuronal activity of a particular type and in particular parts of the central nervous system. These effectors also require that other parts of the nervous system be quiescent. Looking at it from this angle, we may come to the conclusion that the effectors of qualia are very similar in their neuronal bases to the neuronal bases of motor FAPs—except that they appear to be internalized FAPs. Internally, motor FAPs are silent in terms of expression until they are liberated into action; the outward expression of this is a stereotypical movement. By contrast, what I shall refer to as sensory FAPs find their endpoint or overt expression *internally;* this expression is what we call subjective experience. Sensory FAPs are accompanied by subjective experience whether they are produced by activation from stimuli of the external world via our sensory systems, by direct, experimental electrical (or chemical) stimulation of various areas of the brain, or through internally derived activation, as in dreams. It is quite clear that sensory components evoked by direct experimental activation of the brain mostly produce small fragments of sensation rather than the complete sensory events that are generated by normal, physiological activation of the brain. This is not surprising. Compared to the normal physiological activation of the brain, with the complex intricacies of its electrical detail, exogenously applied electrical stimulation must be extraordinarily gross at best, limited in its articulation, range of effect, and the like.

We can demonstrate that electrical stimulation of a certain brain area produces a sensation and that disruption of the electrical activity within or leading to the same area is accompanied by a disappearance of such sensations. Thus we can say again that qualia most certainly relate to electrical activity and location. At this point there are a few possible scenarios that we can consider. One, as many people believe, is that qualia represent a very profound event in neuronal function dealing with quantum mechanical structures of neurons that include the detailed organization of microtubules and microfilaments. This of course opens up a new, previously unexplored area of neuroscience that I won't explore here, for I sincerely doubt it is a plausible scenario worth pursuing at any serious level. The reason for its dismissal is that the neuronal elements that support sensory activation seem to be quite similar to those that support motor activity. Qualia seem to be related not only to particular neurons per se, but also more to the geometrical, electrical patterns of activity neurons are capable of supporting.

To me the evolutionary reason for qualia is straightforward. Qualia represent an ultimate bottom line, because sensations themselves are geometric, electrically triggered events. At this time we cannot reduce it any further. If this geometric, functional state is sensation itself, a serious philosophical problem immediately arises. By this definition are not qualia just another example of "that which we have yet to understand"? Or are they perhaps something of a qualitatively different character altogether, something transcending the neurological substrate of neurons and their electrical activity we attempt to hide them behind? I don't think so, for I believe that patterned electrical activity in neurons and their molecular counterparts are sensations.

"The Hard Problem": Is It True that Science Will Never Understand Feelings?

So, as for the neurobiological basis of qualia, one could leave the issue at the level of the observation that qualia are functional electrobiological events supported by particular sets of neuronal circuits and related to the activation of some neurons and the silence of others within such a network. While this basic description may appear trite it is the only possible basis for a scientific approach to this problem. Ultimately, we will need to know much more about the intricate workings of the nervous system before we can begin to understand what feelings are all about. However, what can we say about qualia today?

For all intents and purposes, the question of qualia or feelings is the question of conscious experience. The feasibility of our ever understanding such an elusive phenomenon in scientific terms is a subject of continuous debate—even as to whether any hypothetical explanation grounded in physical/neural processes can be fully satisfying and complete (see Chalmers 1995, 1997; Shear 1997, for a discussion of various approaches to this issue). While an answer to these questions may be inaccessible at the present time, we can at least attempt to frame the question in a useful way.

David Chalmers, one of the prominent recent voices in this debate, sets up the problem by first noting that consciousness is an ambiguous term that has been used to refer to a collection of distinguishable phenomena, including what he terms the "easy problems" and also the "hard problem" of conscious experience itself:

The easy problems of consciousness are those that seem directly susceptible to the standard methods of cognitive science, whereby a phenomenon is explained in terms of computational or neural mechanisms. The hard problems are those that seem to resist those methods. The easy problems of consciousness include those of explaining the following phenomena:

the ability to discriminate, categorize, and react to environmental stimuli;
the integration of information by a cognitive system;
the reportability of mental states;
the ability of a system to access its own internal states;

the focus of attention;
the deliberate control of behavior;
the difference between wakefulness and sleep. (Chalmers 1995)

and:

For these phenomena, once we have explained how the relevant functions are performed, we have explained what needs to be explained. The hard problem, by contrast, is not a problem about how functions are performed. For any given function that we explain, it remains a nontrivial further question: why is the performance of this function associated with conscious experience? The sort of functional explanation that is suited to answering the easy problems is therefore not automatically suited to answering the hard problem. (Chalmers 1997)

Chalmers collects all these "easy" phenomena associated with consciousness under the umbrella term "awareness" (functional, reportable phenomena), and then argues that there is an inextricable linkage between awareness and experience, almost as cause and effect:

To a first approximation, the contents of awareness are the contents that are directly accessible and potentially reportable, at least in a language-using system.

Awareness is a purely functional notion, but it is nevertheless intimately linked to conscious experience. In familiar cases, wherever we find consciousness, we find awareness. Wherever there is conscious experience, there is some corresponding information in the cognitive system that is available in the control of behavior, and available for verbal report. Conversely, it seems that whenever information is available for report and for global control, there is a corresponding conscious experience. Thus, there is a direct correspondence between consciousness and awareness. (Chalmers 1995)

We return to the essential issue as Chalmers roots this mapping of awareness to conscious experience within the physical mechanisms of the brain:

In general, any information that is consciously experienced will also be cognitively represented. . . . This principle reflects the central fact that even though cognitive processes do not conceptually entail facts about conscious experience, consciousness and cognition do not float free of one another but cohere in an intimate way. (Chalmers 1995)

The linkage Chalmers provides us may be correct, but it may also be secondary to the fundamental origin of qualia as arising from the very properties of physical mechanisms present in the living organism, and more ancient than the cognitive processing of a complex brain. Cause and effect driven from the other end, at least conceptually. In this regard,

I feel there is a possible hypothesis that can be offered concerning the very nature of qualia. This view may be considered as coming from left field, so let me prepare the scenario just a bit.

We have known for a long time that single cells are capable of irritability, that is, the ability to respond to stimuli with a behavioral response consisting of either moving away from, or approaching an object or another cell. In the latter case the relation may be that of hunting for food or fleeing from deleterious or threatening conditions. These observations should remind us that there are in single cells certain abilities related in a primitive way to intentionality, and thus to what may be considered a primitive sensory function. If we are allowed to consider that qualia *represent a specialization of such primitive sensorium,* then it is a reasonable conceptual journey from there to the multicellular phenomenon of "corporate feelings" manifested by higher organisms. If this is something we can live with, then we will understand that *qualia must arise from, fundamentally, properties of single cells* (figure 10.2), amplified by the organization of circuits specialized in sensory functions.

This means that only those circuits having the necessary numbers of sensory cells organized with a particular architecture will be able to support such a function. This can be seen with muscle cells, where the contractile property that characterizes each one is nothing other than a specialization of filamentous interactions found in all cells, a specialization prominent because of architecture. In muscles, actin and myosin molecules are organized parallel to each other to support the sliding filament network and are also anchored to the endoskeletal system, so the force generated by interaction among filaments may add vectorially to support cell contraction (Huxley 1980). If many cells can sum the force generated by their simultaneous contraction, in this case by converging on to a common point (a tendon), then a macroscopic force capable of producing movement is generated. A corporate motor has been evolved. Something similar may be happening with sensory cells. Their summing properties can and have been studied, as we will see presently. That which is summed (single cell primitive qualia-like property) is what must be understood, but the problem then seems far more tractable. We are not searching for a spook.

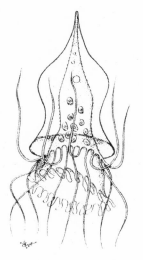

Figure 10.2
Drawing of the one-celled organism *Codonella companella,* illustrating the high degree of structural specialization possible in a single cell. (From Villee-Dethier, 1971, figure 3-2, p. 33.)

The Issue of Qualia as a Single-Cell Property

So what can we say concerning the role of single cells in the generation of qualia? The simplest way to address the issue is to consider other cellular properties that might be, even remotely, related to the problem at hand. What other systems do we know in which electrical signaling is the trigger for coherent cell action? The best analog may be, as mentioned before, muscle contraction.

The following properties are common for muscle contraction and qualia:

1. They are both triggered by electrical activation of the cell.
2. In both, the cellular event of interest is separable from the electrical event that triggers it, and follows in time the electrical activation.

3. The "corporate event" of muscle contraction or qualia has summing properties relating to the numbers of elements activated and to the frequency of activation.

• In muscle the product of cellular activation, force, is the *sum (linear)* of the pull of each cell, onto a common tendon (a geometric property) *at a given time.*

• In qualia the product of cellular activation "sensation" is the *sum (logarithmic)* of each cell activation on to a common coherent event (a geometric property), *at a given time.*

4. Drugs can affect muscle contraction and qualia.

• Modification of electrical activity by sodium conductance block (e.g., TTX) will prevent both muscle contraction and qualia.

• Drugs can modulate muscle contraction by acting on membrane receptors that modify particular molecular events inside the cell (glibencamide) (Light et al. 1994). Similarly, drugs can modulate qualia by acting on membrane receptors that modify particular molecular events inside the cell (psychotropic drugs like marijuana).

The following properties are different as they relate to muscle contraction and qualia:

1. In muscle contraction and qualia the ultimate products are quite different.

• Force is an old physical concept that relates fundamentally to the rapid exchange of virtual force carrying particles among molecules inside the muscle cell (sliding filament theory).

• Qualia (subjective sensation) is an old "natural philosophy" concept that relates fundamentally to nothing that we know about at this moment, inside a cell.

2. Muscle cells are easily recognizable by their very specific internal structure. Neurons that may support qualia are not presently distinguishable in form from those that do not. What is more, it is not clear that there are any differences, at this time.

3. Muscle cells can contract in in vitro conditions. Sensory neurons cannot be demonstrated to generate qualia in conditions other than in an intact animal. Thus electrical stimulation of neurons may generate a sensation as reported by a behavioral response such as the statement "yes I felt that" from a human.

Note that the similarities outweigh the differences and that the areas of difference belong to a single category, lack of specific knowledge.

Can Qualia Be Quantified?

If the brain attempts at all times to decrease the functional overhead of motor control, it is difficult to believe that it does not do the same for sensory systems. So of what are qualia a simplification? We cannot experience everything all at once, all the time, so qualia provide a construct based on what the thalamocortical system deems worthy on a moment-to-moment basis of focus/attention/significance.

Is there a particular way in which perception, through any sense modality, can be understood to work? Is there an underlying pattern that can give us some insight into the functional architecture supporting qualia? In other words, is there a measure for qualia that illuminates the nature of the functional architecture that stages qualia? There is. The measure *for all qualia* can be given mathematically by the Weber-Fechner law (Cope 1976), governing the relationship between the intensity of sensory activation and perception:

$$s = k\ln A/A_o$$

Where s is sensory experience, k is a proportionality constant, ln is the natural logarithm, and A is sensory activation. A_o is the level of sensory activation at which there is no sensory experience; that is, the stimulus remains just under the threshold of perception. One can see that as the amplitude of A increases, the sensory experience increases in a constant ratio, in a geometrical progression based on the value of e, 2.17, the base for the natural logarithm.

We may intuit quite easily this mathematical progression that divides sensory experience into discretely perceived events in terms of musical pitch. Perceptual differences in pitch are detected by humans in steps as small as a few thousandths of a percent change in sound frequency. If we look at musical notation, we realize that the notes corresponding to given increments (or decrements) in sound frequency have a certain proportional change from a center point frequency, or interval. For example, an octave corresponds to twice the frequency of this center sound, and so the increase in the octave frequency corresponds to twice for the next octave, four times for two octaves up, eight times for three, and so on regardless of which note we choose to start with. Likewise, the musical staff, the five parallel, horizontal lines used in musical notation since Guido de Arezzo introduced this system 1000 years ago, denotes the logarithm of sound frequency expressed vertically, with time denoted from left to right (figure 10.3). In fact, ethnomusicologists recognize that the seven basic note structure of the Western system is by no means unique. The notes of the Indian musical system, sa, ri, ga, ma, pa, dha and ni, are identical in every respect to the do, re, mi, fa, sol, la, si, notes of the Western system. It may be more than a coincidence that we also recognize seven colors; the structure of the seven color bands of a rainbow is constant to our qualia. The order is always the same; the thickness is of a certain type. This suggests that the number seven plays perhaps an important, pervasive demarcating role in sensory experience; this is supported by the thesis, "seven, plus or minus two," the magic number that George Miller has so elegantly described.

With respect to this geometry, I think the basic structure of qualia most likely consists of a center point for any sensory experience, with a number of levels above and below as ratios of the central value (two to four levels in systems based on five to nine primary points, respectively). By center point I refer to the level at which most receptors for a given sense modality operate, their most common firing rate or pattern. Firing rates above or below this central point would trigger a modulation back toward it. If one thinks of body temperature, the center point around which the system operates is 36.5 degrees Celsius. Shifting above or below this value sets into motion events that will bring the system back to its naturally selected set point. Similarly, in the human vestibular system, the system that manages our sense of balance, the center point of neural activity is based on the body being upright and erect. The vestibular neurons that fire most frequently do so during the least amount of body movement, indicating the importance of being upright as the center point for balance to operate around.

In considering how a functional geometry such as this may have come to be, it is worth noting that natural growth, when unimpeded, occurs at the logarithmic base e, as described by John Napier in 1614. This universal constant, the solution to $\ln x = 1$, rules all growth (see Thompson, *On*

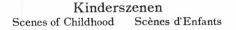

Kinderszenen
Scenes of Childhood   Scènes d'Enfants

Robert Schumann, Op.15
Komponiert 1838

Von fremden Ländern und Menschen
From foreign Lands and People   Hommes et pays nouveaux

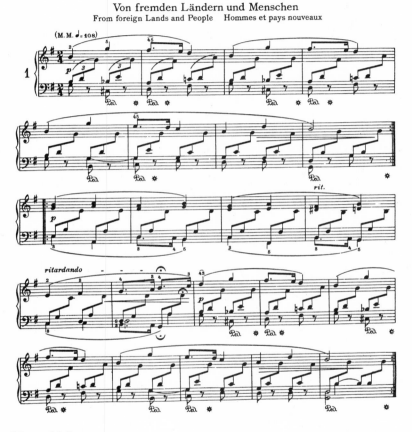

Figure 10.3
Musical notation illustrating the seven-tone western music system. As illustrated in this famous piano composition by Robert Schumann, the pitch of each note is specified by its position on the treble (top) or bass (bottom) clef.

Growth and Form), and is wonderfully evident in the shell curvature of the mollusk *Nautilus,* which exemplifies one of the beautiful and ubiquitous geometric structure in nature. It would not be surprising to find that qualia derive from electrical architectures embedded in neuronal circuits capable of such logarithmic order. If sensations conform to the geometry described by the Weber-Fechner law, it seems quite possible that the electrical patterns of neurons that represent qualia would operate on a similar, logarithmically geometric basis.

So What Are Qualia Good For?

Given our knowledge today, we seem to have come as close as we can to understanding qualia. Those who reject the reduction of qualia to the electrical activity and geometry of neuronal circuits perhaps do so because they lack any understanding of functional geometries; qualia are not some mysterious events that, "residing between," manage miraculously to change the nature of electrical activity into "feelings." After all, we must remember that, as stated above, *qualia are soluble in local anesthetics.* Here the ghost in the machine is responsive to surgery or even a whack on the head. Since when are transcendent properties so fragile and close to the biological process? Parsimony and serious science clearly indicate that "the bridge," "the mysterious transformation" of electrochemical events into sensations is an empty set. It does not exist: neuronal activity and sensation are one and the same event.

Indeed, if a single cell is not capable of having a modicum of qualia, how then can a group of cells generate something that does not belong to a given individual? We would have to say that asking if qualia are properties of a single cell is similar to asking if movement is a property of a single cell. As stated above, movement, as in the case of a limb, is produced by the summed contractile properties of many muscle cells. A single muscle cell cannot produce macroscopical movement of a limb. To follow the argument through, nerve cells must be capable of a "protoqualia." An organized sensation requires the activation of many neurons in a particular pattern, that is, it requires the generation of a neuronal architecture capable of supporting macroscopic qualia in the same way that the musculoskeletal apparatus requires a certain architecture to produce movement.

Coming back to the issue of sensory FAPs, there is a concept that has been lurking in the halls of neuroscience about as long as that discipline has been around. It is the concept of "labeled lines," and it may further help us theoretically remove the ghost in the machine once and for all. The concept of labeled lines states that sensory pathways of all sense modalities encode the specific properties of the world they convey by very specific firing patterns, and that each line or pathway only carries information of that specific modality. In literal terms, these specific patterns *are* the specific sense modality messages from the outside world.

It makes intuitive sense that the perception of high frequency sound requires receptors that convert sound waves into neural energy. These are the hair cells of the auditory apparatus, which respond to high frequency sound with a correspondingly high rate of firing. Similarly, hair cells respond with a low rate of firing when presented with low-frequency sound. Pacinian corpuscles, receptors of the skin that respond to mechanical compression, fire their labeled line message of low frequency pulsing in response to light compression of the skin, and correspondingly higher frequencies of firing for increased mechanical compression. And so it is that the initial message carried by a given sensory pathway faithfully "labels" its outer world counterpart. This frequency coding property, and the fact that each sensory pathway only carries information about its specific sense modality, has led to the concept of labeled lines.

But let us follow one of these labeled lines a little farther, right into the central nervous system. The high frequency firing of the auditory apparatus in response to sound of high frequency does not remain as such. As we follow this labeled line, the high frequency activity is translated into *low* frequency activity by the time it reaches its end point (auditory cortical neurons). This tells us something very important: it is not the code or message coming from the outside world that is being transmitted, but rather it is the neuronal element that responds to the message from the outside that is *itself* the message! It is the sensation born of an internally activated sensory FAP—one may justifiably say that the labeled line carries de facto the frequency because it fired!

Are we getting any closer to a definable functional architecture for qualia? Let us pursue a bit further this concept of the effectors of sensation as being sensory FAPs. From what we learned in chapters 2 and 7, we came to understand that motor FAPs represent a naturally selected functional organization of the central nervous system, one slanted toward computational efficiency. These "plug and play" modules, when activated or released, automatically call to order the various muscle groups and synergies required for a stereotypical movement execution, from the simple to the complex. The computational efficiency, the reader will recall, is attained by the preset automaticity of these modules of function: the brain does not have to reinvent the wheel, from a neuronal circuit (connectivity) perspective, each and every time a particular routine movement is required of the body by circumstance. This allows the central nervous system to put its mind to other things, so to speak. The effectors of FAPs are the motor neurons and the muscles whose contractions the motor neurons drive. Put another way, generated from the internal functional geometry within the basal ganglia is a translation into expression through the functional geometry of how the body can and needs to move, given the momentary (internal and/or external) context.

Can we think of qualia—sensations or sensory experience—in the same way? We can, and the key here is the brain's innate drive toward reducing overhead. A few moments ago I spoke of high-frequency auditory signals being translated to low-frequency activity once this sensory pathway enters more deeply into the central nervous system; this is quite consistent with what we have been saying about an economy of transmission. Rather than the elements being generated from simple to complex, each element carries its own significance and the whole is assembled by the pre-existent presence of significant activity and the absence of other significant activity.

This point is right in line with what we came to understand about the functional organization of sensory systems described in chapter 5. By the very nature of the translation of the geometry of the properties of the external world into the geometry of the internal functional space, reality is at all times *simplified*. It has to be so; it is the only way the brain can keep up with reality. It must simplify at all times.

The Necessity for Qualia

Why is it so important to address the question of qualia in animals? Most people are apparently not convinced that qualia are necessary for any animal. One could, it is supposed, perform exactly the same actions without qualia or feelings. Life would be exactly the same without it! A cat could do everything it does as an automation without qualia: there is no added advantage, there is no reason to have qualia. Should we then deny the fact that they exist? To me, by contrast, qualia, from the perspective of the workings of the brain, constitute the *ultimate* bottom line. Qualia are that part of self that relates (back) to us! *It is a fantastic trick!* One cannot operate without qualia; they are properties of mind of monumental importance. Qualia facilitate the operation of the nervous system by providing well-defined frameworks, the simplifying patterns that implement and increase the speed of decision and allow such decisions to re-enter (the system) and become part of the landscape of perception. Not only were you pricked on the side by the thorn and you moved, but now you have also been sensitized to thorns in general—you can either stay away from them or you can *tame* them, that is, use them as weapons. And so, qualia become exceedingly important tools in perceptual integration; it is the repository of the binding event.

In chapter 5 we took a closer look at the evolution of the eye and saw that nature generates very complex functional architectures. Along with the eye, the heart, and so on, FAPs and even language may be considered as organs, local modules of function with very specialized capabilities and duties. We may, and I think we *must* come to understand qualia as a sort of master organ, one that allows for the individual senses to operate or co-mingle in an ensemble fashion. Qualia make simplifying, momentary judgements about this ensemble activity, allowing these judgements to be re-entered into the system for the predictive needs of the organism (self). Qualia represent judgements or assessments at the circuit level of the information carried by sensory pathways, or sensations. And these sensations, the integration product of the activation of internal sensory FAPs, represent the ultimate predictive vectors that recycle/re-enter into the internal landscape of the self. They *are* the "ghost" in the machine and represent the critically important space between input and output, for they are neither, yet are a product of one and the drive for the other. And all the while they are simplified constructs on the part of the intrinsic properties of the neuronal circuits of our brains.

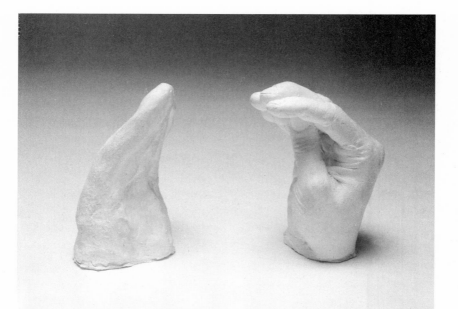

Kiki Smith, *Tongue and Hand*, 1985. Painted plaster, 5-1/2 × 3-1/2 × 3″ (14 × 8.9 × 7.6 cm) tongue unit; 5-1/2 × 3 × 3-1/2″ (14 × 7.7 × 8.9 cm) hand unit. Photograph by Ellen Page Wilson. Courtesy of PaceWildenstein.

11

Language as the Child of
Abstract Thought

The Beginnings of Abstraction

Let us begin by agreeing on a consensus definition of abstraction and/or
abstract thinking. An abstraction generally refers to something that only
exists in the mind: an idea, a conception, a mental representation of
something that may (or may not) exist in the outside world. Abstraction,
or the collection of neural processes that generate abstraction, is a fundamental principle of nervous system function. The nature of these processes owes its origin to the phylogenetic wiring patterns acquired by the
nervous system on its evolutionary course. As such, it is more than likely
that abstract thinking probably began long ago in very primitive nervous
systems. This view emerges from considering the nervous system as being
geared toward predictive movement. In order to place movement within
the context of the whole animal, the animal must first be capable of generating some type of internal "image" or description of itself as a whole,
and this image must support the strategy around which to organize the
tactics of what the animal will do.

At first glance, the generation of a voluntary internal sensory-motor
transformation (see chapter 7) does not correspond directly to the more
obvious neuronal connectivity required to transform, for example, a

stubbing of the toe into a leg flexion. The newer type of wiring represents more than the segmental reflex. It is metasegmental, representing a global function such as the coordinated walking of an elongated multisegmental animal rather than just the stepping supported by a given local segment. By "elongated animal," I refer to any encephalized creature with a head end and a tail or foot end with a column or chain of nervous tissue traversing (and subserving) the length of the body. This description encompasses a broad range from the more lowly creatures with very primitive notochords to those with quite sophisticated spinal cords. That the nervous system was selected in evolution to be organized in a segmented fashion was probably driven by the neurobiological practicality of optimizing body surface area to volume, in order to minimize the distance a nerve signal must travel either to or from the external world. Elongated animals are basically made of a horizontal stack of "coins," where the neural wherewithal subserving each coin is organized to know about its respective segment and relatively little else. In order to make a complete working animal out of these segments, there *must* be a portion of the nervous system that is *not* exclusively segmental in its organization. This portion of the nervous system can put the many segments together into something that beforehand did not exist: a unified whole. As stated above, we may consider this the beginning of abstract function as this portion of the nervous system does not relate *directly* to the connectivity of the nervous system at any particular, segmental level. The central nervous system abstracts the fact that the animal is composed of a series of unit segments; ipso facto, the process of intersegmental integration is an abstraction, and represents the beginning of abstraction as a naturally selected biological process. That this is the evolutionary direction is supported by the observation that the central nervous system mushrooms out in front of the spinal cord, polarizing encephalization. We see something important happening: from the animal's very neurological becoming is the fact that the animal can have an internal *representation* of itself not only as a set of parts but as a whole entity. It is here, from this germinal metaevent, that abstraction begins and the self emerges.

How does this relate to prediction? Well, beyond the description of the animal itself and the description of the input that comes to this animal, the intrinsic circuits of the nervous system are capable of generating a premotor representation of what is going on outside. From this, self-referentially in the presence of that motor image, the animal is capable of deciding what to do. The animal is capable of prediction. Run, fight, find food or whatever, functionally the animal *is* the circuit that represents its sensory motor attributes, and this central event is an abstract entity.

Now of great importance is the event that happens between the stimulus that evokes movement and the liberated motor FAP. The prompting stimulus may be of external origin (a ferret is climbing up my pants!) or internal (I left the stove on at home!). Either way, these stimuli, if granted appropriate internal significance (by and within the momentary status or context of the cycling thalamocortical system), are amplified into an emotional state. We have already seen that the nervous system is wired in such a way that under normal conditions FAPs are only liberated into action by the generated emotional states that precede them. Such internal events, emotions, are then by definition premotor states.

We can take this further. Emotions or emotional states are events that do not exist in the outside world; they are purely internal events and would remain completely hidden to us (as observers of others) were it not for motricity. Precisely *which* emotion may be occurring is inferred only through the expression of the FAP that is liberated by that given emotion. The dog is snarling and baring its teeth at me; what is going on inside of this dog is most likely not that he is happy to see me. Just how it is that I came to know or infer this is another important issue that we will discuss shortly. The point here is that emotions, being themselves purely internal events, are simply invented states on the part of the central nervous system and as such are clearly abstractions. It is fair to say that just as emotions are intrinsic products of central nervous system function, so are abstractions.

Intentionality

Returning to prediction, it is clear that prediction must have a goal, otherwise it is not referentially based on anything; purposeless movement is not only wasteful, but can be quite dangerous as well. The goal or object of movement must be well defined, and we may define it here as that which one intends to do *in relation to* that object or goal. Also an abstraction, intentionality is the premotor detail of the desired result of movement through which a particular emotional state is expressed: the choice of what to do before the doing of it.

Consider the following: if our brains are capable of planning movement strategies that are implementable if desired, then they should also be able to outwardly express *intentionality* as a motor representation of what is happening inside our heads. I am suggesting that the outward expression of *premotor* activity precedes and predicts the activation of specific motor patterns. An example of such a process is shouting "run!" when in danger before we actually begin to run. This raises a crucially important point about language itself. I suggest that our ability to vocalize the different aspects of intentionality developed first *as the ability to separate the properties of things from the things themselves.* This process of abstraction would over time engender what we may consider to be a mental catalog, much like an alphabet, that would allow us to generate inside our heads events that would be reentered admixtures of the primary events that went into the generation of language to begin with. We have arrived at our first corollary: even before language was sufficiently well structured to be communicable, its genesis must have had as a prerequisite foundation the nervous system's capacity to generate the premotor imagery required to abstract the properties of things from the things themselves. That is, it required the premotor imagery to make abstractions of universals.

And so we see that there are two very important issues we must bear in mind when considering the evolution of language. One, that abstract thinking must have preceded language during evolution, and two, that the premotor events leading to expression of language are in every way the same as those premotor events that precede any movement that is executed for a purpose. From these two points, which are so similar as to be almost the same, we may gather that language is simply an element within a much larger, more general category of function.

Prosody: The First Cracklings of Language

Let us now dig into the plausible origins of language and how this indispensable tool must have evolved. Just as in the case of the rather meandering evolution of the eye, language may be difficult to trace cleanly backwards through evolutionary time (see, for discussions and concepts, MacNeilage 1994, 1998; Verhaegen 1995; Gordon 1996; Ujhelyi 1996; Aboitiz and Garcia 1997 a, b; Honda and Kusakawa 1997; Ganger and Stromswold 1998; Gannon et al. 1998; Kay et al. 1998; Doupe and Kuhl 1999; Nowak and Krakauer 1999). As in previous examples, evolutionary steps prior to the emergence of a specialized organ may not necessarily function or appear in any fashion similar to what we see in the present day organ. As we learned from the lifetime of lifetimes that brought us the eye, we may perhaps expect an unexpected genealogical path in the ancestry of language.

Now before proceeding further, we must gather a few clarifying definitions. Just what do we mean by "language"? The first thing that typically comes to mind is human language, its wide variety of types, that it is often written as well as spoken, and that languages other than our own are at once fascinating and opaque. If you feel that language is exclusively a human capability or that we humans invented language, then I must tell you that I wholeheartedly disagree, although you may not be alone in this thinking. The reasons for which I disagree are straightforward: language clearly exists in many species far, far older in the evolutionary sense than we *Homo sapiens;* furthermore it is too general a trait throughout the animal kingdom ever to be seriously considered as exclusive to humans. Although it is most likely true that we exhibit the richest and most complex of languages, we are neither the origin nor sole possessor of language.

Let us define language as the given methodology by which one animal may communicate with another. In this regard, language is a rather large, generic category, for this definition says nothing about the *intent* to communicate, only that some level of communication is ultimately achieved. We have so far been saying that language is a logical product of the intrinsic abstracting properties of the central nervous system, or simply of abstract thought. But this I would say is a subcategory within language that I would call biological "prosody." Prosody is a more generalized form of motor behavior, an outward gesturing of an internal state, an outward expression of a centrally generated abstraction *that means something to another animal.* For us, smiling, laughter, frowning, the lifting of one's eyebrows are all forms of prosody, for they convey one's internal, momentary state in a way that is recognizable and understandable to someone else. Prosody is language, but it is not spoken language. Nonetheless, it is purposeful communication. Prosody is by no means confined to humans; it is widespread throughout the animal kingdom, and in the evolutionary sense is very old. Darwin, in his brilliant text on facial expression, studied prosody in animals in terms of moods and faces and how faces and postures represent the momentary internal states of an animal. These are representations of the internal abstractions such as emotions and intentions. So a prosodic event is an abstraction coupled with a motor expression that conveys to another animal what its internal state is like at that moment.

If prosody represents a subcategory within language, what would be an example of language *without* prosody? Well, there are types of language that are extraordinarily specific and although they carry very simple messages, they are nevertheless essential for the survival of the species. The pheromone delivery and reception systems of a moth are known to be effective for distances of several miles, and so they clearly represent communication at a distance. The pheromone released by the female is recognized specifically and exclusively by the male of the same species and is communicatively effective enough for the couple to find each other in an otherwise crowded niche (Willis and Arbas 1991; Hildebrand 1995; Roelofs 1995; Baker et al. 1998). But although this language is critical for the species' survival, it has nothing to do with the outward expression of an internally generated abstraction. This is therefore not prosody, but rather simply a behavior-modifying event through the release and reception of a specific molecule.

In most cases, however, language circumscribes a prosodic event. We find that language as such may be observed at many levels in evolution, where it serves very different functions. One of the first nonhuman languages to be understood sufficiently by people, one that communicates simple orders, is the language of bees. This language is basically a dance, a rhythm and orientation performed in space. These dances, each one specific to bees of a particular species, give information about the quantity and location of food with respect to the beehive. In this way all bees of the colony can know about and help procure the food (von Frisch 1994; Gould 1976, 1990; Hammer and Menzel 1995; Menzel and Muller 1996; Waddington et al. 1998). Languages such as these have also been studied in vertebrates and other invertebrates. By definition and in all cases, these forms of communication require social order so that the information conveyed may be used to some purpose by the receiving organism.

There are variations of language that convey information quite different from just the issue of food for one's family. For instance, when most animals are attacked, they generally posture in a manner that is clearly recognizable as a defensive stance by the attacker or as a counter-punch ready to occur. Such posturing may be as simple as a puffer fish increasing its size to appear more formidable, or the very common showing of teeth and growling we see in most vertebrates. Animals with horns, such as the rhinoceros or buffalo, take a stance where the horns are directed at the threatening or attacking animal. These are all languages, granted with very limited repertoire, but this form of prosody must be at the very foundation of all types of purposeful communication between and within species.

Moving higher up the evolutionary scale, we can look at languages that convey a higher level of organization. The language of wolves is an excellent example where by means of prosody, wolf packs express relatively complex, socially structured attack and defense behaviors. In this case, the relations between the differing animals are not only of simple prosody but also represent a (social) context within which this prosodic language is exercised.

This form of prosody in wolves is quite sophisticated, utilizing a number of different motor avenues for overall expression, including vocalization, eye contact, head gesturing, and whole body communication. For instance, the establishment of dominance, or which wolf is to be the alpha male, is by means of communication not just of one's physical might, but by those males subordinate to the alpha male showing their social position by expressing submission. They will roll over onto their backs and offer the alpha male their neck. This form of language leads to an establishment of social hierarchy that is central to the strategies of the pack as a whole. However, during hunting other factors arise, and so:

True leadership is not strongly apparent in a wolf pack, as any animal may initiate its movement. However, the pack is highly cooperative in hunting and in the care of the young. Dominance organization is not strongly apparent in wild wolf packs, but in the captive packs in zoos, where the principle occupation of hunting is made unnecessary by artificial feeding, wolves spend a large amount of their time threatening one another and enforcing dominance. (Dewsbury and Rethlingshafer, 1973)

Notwithstanding this caution about the risks of using behavior observed in captivity to make sweeping generalizations about behavior in the wild, the social organization of wolves does have a hierarchy, so the language or the prosodic events would be understood differently at its different levels. The prosody that cues one adult male to know that it is his turn within an attack sequence may to a young pup be simply the learning of the global differences between attacking and defending. The main point here is that the social hierarchy itself could not exist of there were no elements of commonality existing at all levels. In this case we see that language is developed in the context of a particular social order as a means of binding animals into a single working entity for the benefit of all.

Similarly, there are very interesting hunting behaviors that one sees in wild dogs of Africa. They often attack where there is tall grass, for that is usually where the smaller animals of prey are found. These dogs have white-tipped tails that they keep straight up in the air. They move their tails back and forth in particular patterns that stimulate peripheral vision, so each dog, without having to look around that much, can see where the other tails are, and thus receive a constantly updated status report on the structure of the pack as it flushes out and/or corners its prey. It is fascinating to ponder here the reasonable conclusion that anatomy has evolved to be related to the language of *strategy*.

These prosodic, ensemble properties of the canine species have made possible the very particular relationship that dogs have with man. This relation is especially clear in situations where dog and man form a working team, as in shepherding or hunting. Here the dog is simply expressing properties (abstraction and prosody) that were genetically determined and is imprinting the relations of the hierarchy it already knows—save for the fact that here, the hierarchy is with an animal other than another dog.

Mimicry: The Origin of Meaning Between Organisms

What seems to be emerging is that language must have evolved from a prelinguistic type of attribute, mostly concerning prosody, punctuated by either particular sounds or particular gestures. But we must not overlook a very crucial element to language. If prosody is the outward expression of a momentary internal state, what is its purpose unless it is understood by another animal? Communication without consensus meaning simply is not communication. So what we are really asking is: How did the meaning part come to communication?

Here is something I would have to refer to as the infectious nature of brain activity. Laughter is the perfect example—it is infectious between people. Someone begins laughing, you hear (and/or see) this, and soon you cannot help but laugh. Put another way, laughter is generated and when you receive it, *you create the similar state in your head*. It is as if the abstraction itself is infectious—an intrinsic property of neuronal circuits that seems to get outside of itself. We may think that if laughter in infectious, and so is yawning, then maybe showing your teeth and growling is infectious as well. Let's examine this point further.

Consider the kookaburra, a bird of Australia. These birds hang out together, usually spotting the branches of two or three neighboring trees. From the silence, one of the birds starts making the characteristic kookaburra sound, which happens to sound, to us, exactly like distorted human laughter. Another kookaburra joins in, mimicking the same sound as the first, and within seconds, the whole flock is "laughing." We see a similar event with fireflies: one male lights up, the others entrain. And so the female, far off in the distance, gets a real *flash!*

What does this mimicry tell us about language? One can imagine that if the nervous system were to acquire by accident the ability to recognize, through sensory input, the FAPs displayed by *others,* this would be a very useful property if the animals are going to live in groups. In fact, this property makes the group *de facto* birds of a feather! And so animals with the ability to mimic each other would immediately tend to form a family, because what has been engendered is indeed a sense of familiarity: Hey! You're one of *us!*

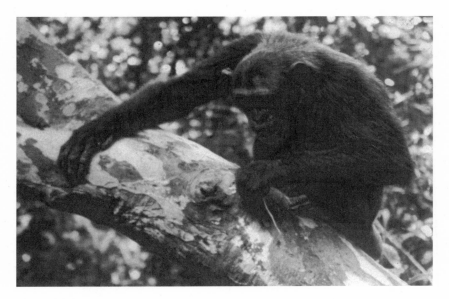

Figure 11.1
Ant fishing learned by mimicry. (Photo by T. Nishida, from Whiten et al. 1999.)

Recognition of one's kin is as old as time. Fair enough, but this recognition is fostered through mimicry, through a creature's repeating the FAPs of others that it gleans through its senses (figure 11.1). But what can one say of communicative meaning across species? I know that the dog still snarling at me from a few pages back means trouble for me. It means trouble to another dog as well. How does it know? How do I know? Rather, how did we *come* to know? Let's wind evolution backward and think it through.

An animal bares its teeth at another animal; the other animal does not recognize this FAP. Nonetheless, this FAP evokes a "show teeth back" or a "run" FAP. Why? Because all of those who didn't at once recognize the baring of teeth FAP *died!* They became lunch, and thus over time they were naturally selected out of the gene pool! But those that remained, in the natural selection sense, evolved to have such FAP recognition become an intrinsic *a priori*. Thus, out of phylogeny comes the ability to recognize certain things as dangerous without necessarily memorizing them in real time, in ontogenetic time. For instance, fish know from birth that very brightly colored (other) fish are dangerous. At birth, they just know it. Those brightly colored fish over there are poisonous; they *advertise* it! And this is as wired as is the fact that fish have tails!

The above is the evolutionary downstream endpoint, if you will, but mimicry is at its origin. Of course we agree that language would make no sense if the receiver did not understand what language means. How does understanding occur? The easiest way for the receiver to understand what language means is for the receiving animal to somehow associate its own production of the motor event with the sensory reception of the motor event. That is, an outward motor expression of the internal sensorimotor image is matched with that which the receiving animal is actually, sensorially, experiencing: monkey see, monkey do. It can be done through learning, but it has to be more powerful than that. It would have to be done by understanding in a sensory way the consequences of this mimicked motor behavior. This is a bit complicated; there is a hurdle to get over.

Let's say I am an alligator now and I bare my teeth. Simple enough, but here's the problem: *I most likely will never see myself baring my teeth*. However, I might hear my own growling and so when a growling occurs I may recognize it as what I do when I am in a certain mood. If I see that growling is often associated with teeth baring I will soon associate the two. This is why when another alligator bares its teeth at me, I don't just ignore it, or simply look the other way as if nothing happened. We are at an evolutionary crux. Coming to know universals must have come from not knowing universals. This can happen in only one of two ways. Either the nervous system absolutely knows in advance what it is doing or it doesn't, in which case it is natural selection that has determined my response: when another alligator bares its teeth at me, I bare mine right back. The answer must be, of course, the latter, natural selection. How do I know? Think of how people act when they see themselves on TV for the first time, or in a film. They are always amazed at how silly they appear to themselves. Something internal does not match with the external presentation of the same event, so just the (sensorimotor image of the) *doing of it* is not enough for a complete understanding. There must be an understanding, in a sensory way, of the consequences of the motor behavior, and the only way is through mimicry: I do not see myself baring my teeth but I know that I do that when I am angry and/or ready to attack. That is my emotional state and that is the FAP it liberates. Now I see this other animal baring its teeth at me: it could be another alligator, or it could be any animal that bares its teeth. Do I put it together that that FAP is the outward expression of the same internal state of anger that I know, or do I not put it together? Hopefully I do put it together—my life depends on it—but the point here is that this is the only way in which an animal can come to recognize and know what the momentary internal state of another animal may be. Furthermore, understanding must be acquired by trial and error and it must be acquired through mimicry, which means attempting to replicate the motor behavior one notices being expressed by another. Such understandings are generalized by trial and error. It may take me forever to understand that a particular gesture by another animal means danger, because I may *not* know that. Instead I may simply have lived around those alligators that do know, long enough, and may simply have mimicked the behaviors displayed by them *after* something bared their teeth and snarled at them. They walked away and so I walk away with them—with not so much as an inkling of an idea as to what the precipitating event might have been! But my chance of survival is increased because I receive the benefits of the knowledge of my fellow alligators. I am naturally selected because I behave as if I know that if something bares its teeth at me it means danger. This is what I mean by the generalization of these understandings and that they too are at the behest of trial and error. We may look at these as providing each animal's specific informational niche, what those around me do and what these things come to mean to me.

It is pattern recognition, of course, but this pattern recognition is totally context-dependent. This is why you can't take an alligator from the Nile and put it in the Amazon and expect it to survive. There is no longer any familiarity of patterns, any matching of the internal with the perceived external. The alligator won't recognize *anything* in its environment, and its system expects a set of external features that are unfortunately completely different from what surrounds it! In other words, abstraction has been bamboozled!

A brief footnote. It appears as if abstraction is seeking a match up of the internal with the external. The system accepts as recognizable patterns that are only close at best, if that. Recall our discussion about imprinting. Clearly this phenomenon employs pattern recognition and thus abstraction to engender and associate understanding or meaning. Another example: recently there has been the creation of an artificial bee from a microchip. It does the dance, communicates with the other, real bees, and off they all race together looking for the food (Montague et al. 1995). And so it doesn't really have to be a bee: just a reasonably close, dynamic, four-dimensional geometric pattern!

Role of Mimicry in Language Development

Let us return to mimicry and its role in the development of language. What routes might natural selection have taken to allow for mimicry to be an intrinsic property? The path of least resistance—what else? We are moving from the ability to mimic to the desire to mimic, a crucial next step. The instinct to mimic is amplified by the fact that for most animals, mimicry is very easily accomplished through the auditory system. Why? Because if you hear a sound you can produce your own sound over and over until it matches. The visual system is more difficult, as I pointed out before, because one usually does not see oneself doing something. So you get mimicry evolving fastest and running rampant in systems where it is very easy for it to flourish.

Mimicry of Sounds

Clearly animals can make sounds. The nice thing about making sounds is that the animal can hear the sounds it makes. The FAP of vocalization makes a huge difference, because the animal can now match from a motor point of view whatever sensory tape it may have, that is, whatever sounds it may be attempting to mimic (remember the bird song issues).

Vocalization is quite a fascinating subject. We tend, for some reason, to lump vocalization and language together, typically in the sense of human language, but vocalization is much older. The true richness of vocalization as we know it evolved once intention or prosody was coupled with that effector. But that effector, vocalization, came first, probably as some motor accident that caused something beneficial and was thus naturally selected for.

Vocalization was itself part of a rather sophisticated FAP to begin with. Which one, you ask? When you hurt, you cry out. And you cry out because it hurts, but this vocalization is also a form of defense. When you cry out you tend to startle for an instant the attacking animal, whether human or other, and this distracts it momentarily from its offensive. If you scream, the attacker may stop and possibly even go away. You have increased your chances of survival. Now think in the evolutionary sense. You scream when you are bitten, when you are attacked. From this it evolves to be that you also may scream when you *think* you are being bitten and/or attacked. Next you simply scream whenever you feel pain, and now it has nothing to do with being attacked. A sharp pang in your stomach, you get a cramp in your leg, you stub your toe on a rock. It generalizes from that.

Vocalizing moves from just representing the responses to external activity to that of *internal* activity. Vocalization is a motor reflection of *arousal*. Now one should not think that arousal is only a response to something from the outside world. To be sure, your alarm clock is a very arousing object. But arousal is an internal state and is generated from within as much as from without. Some hours later you realize that you locked your keys inside your car by mistake: Oh no! This is arousal, absolutely, and this state is generated purely from an internal stimulus, that the concept of locking the keys in the car is a disturbing one. The concept is the stimulus. Or a dream may be so intense that it actually rouses you from sleep. This is again arousal purely from the inside. Stimuli of the external world are beating on the nervous system and stimuli from the internal world are beating on the system; they are in this regard quite equivalent. Thus it is that an animal cries out both because it has been bitten and because it has been bitten from the inside.

And so an animal hears noises, makes noises, hears its own noises being made, and comes to learn what the noises mean when it makes the noise and when it hears another making the (same) noise. This form of mimicry is probably the best way to associate things, as we have said, because when you are angry and you make an angry noise, you will come to recognize as "angry" these noises in other animals. You come to recognize that they are having the same sort of internal experience that you had when you made that particular noise. It is the same as the laughter we spoke of earlier. You come to hear and recognize laughter because you associate it with your own.

Mimicry flourished quite well through these systems because we can hear the sounds we make and make the sounds we hear. If you also possess an apparatus capable of generating sufficiently complex sound and sound patterns, as we have with our sophisticated laryngeal mechanism (Hirose and Gay 1972; Passingham 1981; Doupe 1993; Zhang et al. 1994; Davis et al. 1996; Jurgens and Zwirner 1996; Jurgens 1998; Doupe and Kuhl 1999) and as birds have with their broad-ranged sound shaping syrinx (Goller and Suthers 1996a,b; Goller and Larsen 1997a,b; Wild 1997a,b; Suthers 1997; Suthers et al. 1999), then the complexities of internal meaning and their outward expression will flourish and grow as well. A cow, on the other hand, can "moo," and that's about it; it doesn't have many other voices, so to speak. In humans and many birds, the range of the phonating apparatus is enormous and so naturally becomes selected as a very good medium for communication.

Visual Mimicry

Also quite common in the animal kingdom but not so easy to bring about is mimicry through the visual system. Consider the flounder; although perhaps not the most elegant and beautiful of creatures, the flounder is nonetheless fascinating in its *intent*. Think of a flounder: it has its two eyes on one side of the body, the dark side. The other side, the underbelly, is light colored. A flounder on the bottom of the ocean settles in and disappears into an image of the surrounding external world. What is so intriguing here is that in completing an image of its universe, this particular animal is creating with its body a pattern over a patch of sea bottom that, by definition, it will never see. Its eyes, facing upward, are not positioned to see the terrain the body is covering. The image, made for others to see, is an attempt to mimic the visual context of whatever else is surrounding the fish where it has come to rest. The flounder is creating a pattern in its skin of what the sea floor underneath it *should* look like to others given the surroundings. This is an odd animal. Obviously, if one covers its eyes, it cannot make the (given) pattern. If a flounder is placed on top of a chessboard, it will attempt to copy the pattern to fit in visually and continue the pattern. The important thing is that this fish has to be able to

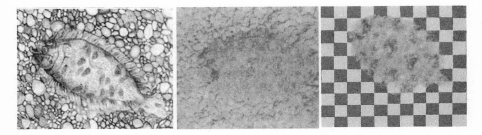

Figure 11.2
Photographs of flounders, illustrating their capacity for camouflaging themselves by changing their appearance to mimic the color and texture of the background. The adaptive changes take place within 2–8 seconds. Left and middle images are of the same fish. (Left from website www.richmond.edu/~ed344/webunits/vertebrates/camouflage.html; middle and right from Ramachandran et al., 1996, figure 1, p. 816.)

generalize, to abstract. It won't manage a great likeness to the chessboard pattern—one can see the clear problems with the optical system of this fish—but it certainly gives it a sporting try. This is a very beautiful case of mimicry from a visual system point of view. The animal has the ability to create a bit of reality that does not exist but that is nonetheless close enough to the terrain for another animal to not be able to discern a discontinuity in what it is seeing (figure 11.2). This camouflaging behavior on the part of the flounder can only be explained by the fact that abstraction must be involved in this type of pattern generation.

Another animal in which we see relatively more evolved mimicry through the visual system is the cuttlefish *Sepia*. These cephalopods have specialized cells in the skin called chromophores that can expand or contract by nervous activation and thus appear to change from white to black (Ferguson et al. 1994; Loi et al. 1996; Shasher et al. 1996). Through the use of the chromophores, the cuttlefish will make all sorts of neonlike patterns, lines and geometries of lines that go this way and that across their bodies. A quite striking effect, this is another example of a probably very complex prosodic language, in this case a purely visual one, a semaphoric type of language, if you will. This is also a very rich language, because the cuttlefish can make these dissipating patterns very rapidly and with a great range of complexity. That there is meaning conveyed by this language between the two animals is clear; from the exactness and speed with which they mimic each other's patterns and the patterns of patterns, it is obvious more is going on than idle reflex. Something must drive the necessary sophistication and control to be able to signal with such an incredible amount of complexity, and that something has *intention to do* written all over it.

Let us summarize briefly. Language must clearly be born of abstraction or abstract thinking, or, to put it another way, the processes generating the abstracting properties of the nervous system must have preceded what we call language, most particularly prosodic language. We have defined prosody as the outward expression of a momentary internal state that by way of this outward expression *means* something to another creature. Such internal states, emotions and intentions alike, do not exist in the outside world and so by definition must be abstractions. How such internal states have come to mean the same thing—or close enough to the same thing to be useful between animals—must have evolved through the conduit of mimicry. Mimicry provides the commonality of same behavior so that the associations between internal states and perceived behavior in others may occur. I do this when I feel this way; I now see you doing this and so maybe you feel the same way when you are doing it. And so, over eons of trial and error, meaning between organisms evolved.

Mimicry has occurred in two primary ways, both of which are reflections of internal abstraction, though of differing types. There is mimicry that is *copying,* such as the "I hear this sound, I make this sound until it matches" method, and there is *extrapolation,* as the flounder does by abstracting itself into a visual pattern that others see. Globally speaking, for meaningful communication, copying sets the stage of commonality by which the nuances of extrapolation may be discerned between creatures.

Of Human Language

From all of the above, it should be clear that language of any kind could not have materialized suddenly out of nowhere, a lightning bolt of advancement in biological evolution. This will not sit well with those who feel that there is no form of true language except for that found in humans, but it is reasonable to consider that abstraction and prosody, whose intra- and interspecies meaning developed slowly out of mimicry, must be the prerequisite elements, the evolutionary preamble, for that which we know as human language.

Language, and in particular human language, arose as an extension of premotor conditions, namely those of the increasing complexities of intentionality as abstract thinking grew richer. It simply became necessary for us humans to do more with what we had, with our motor capabilities, and by increasing the sophistication of purposeful movement through modifying and overriding the existing FAPs. The expansion into a much wider range of motor expression probably occurred at the same time as the ability to override FAPs.

The reader will recall from chapter 7 that the ability to override a liberated FAP is an ability born out of an increasingly elaborate thalamocortical system. It is also most clearly supported by the development of corticospinal connectivity (the so-called pyramidal tract). In a word, we see the addition of increasingly sophisticated intentionality behind purposeful movement. The evolution of such specialized systems as the pyramidal tract, which is related to toe and finger movements, as well as to the activation of the cranial nerves activating lips, tongue, and pharynx-larynx, supported the ability to override particular FAPs, removing inherent constraints. It allowed for the incredible dexterity we see in higher mammals, particularly in simians and humans. It is fair to say that the evolution and enrichment of the cortical mantle, as occurred in the motor system, is the most important overall message to be gathered from the evolution of the cortex. It has been the ability of the nervous system to increase the number of possible functional states without violating the FAPs upon which voluntary movements must ultimately ride. We cannot override FAPs to the point where they simply do not exist or are completely dormant. We have already discussed in depth the critically important need they fill in reducing the nervous system's computational overhead. Rather, it is the finely achieved evolutionary balance between automatic, computational efficiency and the ability to generate necessary nuance to our movements that characterizes our brain as the most exquisitely capable of all brains. These issues are so standard, so taken for granted that we hardly ever realize the incredible coordination of FAPs that is necessary for something so commonplace as giving a public speech. One must be able to maintain an erect, vertical stance, or, perhaps, depending on circumstances, a constant pacing movement, while seamlessly executing the very complicated synergies that allow for respiratory, laryngeal, and orofacial mechanisms to act synchronously to produce even one recognizable word! Add to this prosodic movements such as gesturing with the arms and facial expressions, and we are now describing a rather complex motor event. Yet, for most, it is considered as just walking and talking at the same time.

Let us take the example of the evolution of increased eye/hand coordination, where the new sophistication of cortical connectivity produces a wider variety of possible movements, and yet does so without violating the FAPs that underlie all voluntary movements. We may say here that this new system interlaces with the present FAPs and uses them as columns or buttresses on which to support the very new. Metaphorically speaking, the richer intentionality demands a stage upon which to enact particular plays that have never been played before. This should sound familiar with respect to the processes underlying abstraction, for they are one and the same. In fact, this is precisely where abstract thinking gets particularly purified, as discussed in chapter 6. But, take note, vocalization became with usage a FAP! The new system, bringing increased intentionality and prosodic capabilities, used and expanded the FAP of vocalization, taking advantage of its wide range of (sound) pattern generation. And so, just as the increased complexity of intentionality demanded an increase in the richness of eye/hand coordination, so too did the increased need to express internal abstractions take advantage of and increase the dexterity of the vocal mechanism of the animal. It did so not only with the laryngeal and orofacial structures that shape the different sounds, but also with the entire respiratory apparatus, so necessary in generating the patterned airflow required to make these very specific sounds (Wild 1994; Davis et al. 1996). These sounds, known to us all through the processes of mimicry and repetition, are the phonemes that comprise our language. They represent the very granularity of our language and they are the basis for human language independent of the particular language used. In complicated eye/hand coordination in which the numbers of motor patterns activated are very large (Jeannerod 1986; Miall 1998), the possible patterns are nevertheless finite in number. It is the same with phonemes or the letters of an alphabet: much can be done as these finite grains of motricity become mixed into incredible mosaics of expression. When we add our already rich prosodic capabilities to this language, it is difficult to argue that we, as a species, have evolved to express our internal states more thoroughly than any other species.

With respect to linguistic theory, one major theoretical proposal has been a source of much controversy in this century. This is the concept of modularity as it relates to brain function. As originally stated by Chomsky in his book on the neurological basis of language (Chomsky 1972), it was his view that the unique ability of the human nervous system to generate complex language was produced by a very special function in the brain, probably subserved by a very specialized region. This is not necessarily so. Certainly the presence of Wernicke's area (language comprehension, or auditory association area) and Broca's speech area, and the problems caused by lesions to these areas (alexia, inability to read, anomia, word-finding difficulties, aphasias, speech disorders) provided a strong impetus and justification for this particular view. And yet this answer is unsatisfying, because of the nervous system's limited ability to reorganize itself beyond a certain point, the imprecise localization of these areas, and the possibility of the migration of such functions from one part of the brain to another (for instance as in epilepsy). These findings question the very simplistic view of a phrenological type of modular organization that permeated neurology for many years and that again seemed to be supported by the misuse of noninvasive imaging techniques in what may be called neophrenology. But the fact that it may be difficult to pinpoint a brain event to less than a few cubic centimeters of tissue is not sufficient evidence to discard modularity entirely, especially if such modularity is considered a functional structure, even if a dissipative one.

My own particular reason for accepting this view has to do with patients such as those described in chapter 7 and the issue of FAPs. Not only phonemes but also particular words can be generated by an individual whose brain has been damaged to such an extent that only the most minimal neurological correlate to the module remains (figure 11.3). This indi-

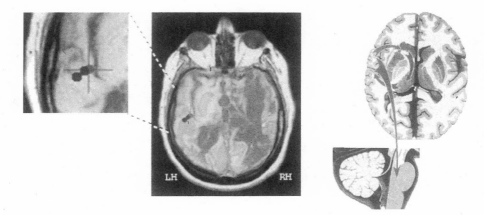

Figure 11.3
Positron emission tomography (PET) scan of a woman who has been in a coma
for more than 20 years in a permanent vegetative state. She spontaneously but infrequently produces isolated words unrelated to any external stimulation. Her
condition developed as a result of a succession of three massive strokes that collectively destroyed all but the basal ganglia, some parts of the thalamus, and a region of the cortex known as Broca's area that controls the motor generation of
speech. The highlighted areas indicate those few brain regions of significant meta-
bolic activity. (See chapter 7, p. 152.) This case history indicates that selected cerebral circuits can support "modular" motor expression. In the case of spoken
words, this requires proper phonological articulation, and the properly timed activation of various muscles (including the diaphragm) in addition to the vocal
cords. (Adapted from Schiff et al. 1999, figure 4).

cates that the motor FAP is necessary and sufficient for the behavior of
that particular module but not sufficient for other aspects of speech, such
as being able to produce the thought required behind the words or even
the appropriate context within which those words should be used.

Jasper Johns, *Gray Alphabets*, 1956. Encaustic on newsprint and pencil on canvas, 168 × 124 cm. © Jasper Johns/Licensed by VAGA, New York, NY. The Menil Collection, Houston.

12 The Collective Mind?

CHAPTER ~~this~~ IS UNCLEAR.

The Issue of Communication

In the last chapter, abstraction was described as an element of a very general category of intrinsic brain function, deriving from the global organization of the nervous system that has been naturally selected for over biological history. As I pointed out, there is a lot of nervous system that does not deal with segmental function. The binding of segmental function into a composite is an abstraction that kinesthetically images the animal as a whole *to itself,* thus affording the animal the ability to place itself in the context of the external world. Further, this evolutionary path of encephalization has as perhaps its most significant characteristic the ever-increasing enrichment of the thalamocortical system, of which we humans are the best and most extreme example. If one were to ask what is the primary benefit of this enrichment, the answer would have to be the ability to override FAPs. When this ability is coupled with the ability to abstract "self," we see in many (relatively higher) animals escape behaviors consisting of complex wriggling movements that help the animal free itself from unexpected problems or from being inadvertently stuck in a constraining position. Such behavior requires that the animal have an image of self within the context of its entrapment, and also that it employ a set of motor solutions to this problem of constraint that go beyond the routine and inadequate FAPs for walking, scratching, or chewing. Consider, for example, the problem faced by an albatross walking about versus flying. The body size and geometry will be totally different, and so different self-images must be deployed.

Both the image of self and the overriding of FAPs demand the use of the abstractive properties of the nervous system. These abstractions escape into the external world, for they may be understood and learned—thus communicated—through mimicry. (If wriggling like that helped my sibling get away, maybe it will help me, too.)

But here we must make an important distinction between ourselves and, say, the squirrel that twists and turns its way loose from a predator. Although the squirrel may show another squirrel or animal that violent jerking and wriggling may help it escape a foe, it cannot *tell* another that this is so. With all due respect to squirrels, the message could be conveyed more effectively with the use of spoken language, which can facilitate the communication of internal abstraction(s), both in detail and accuracy.

Spoken language, as opposed to prosodic body or facial gesturing, in many ways extends the range of communication beyond measure, and also, it extends *the range of the senses*. How? Almost any example will do. A friend stands on my shoulders to look over a very high wall.

"What do you see?" I ask. And he tells me.

Spoken language here clearly allows me to "see" where I cannot.

Or my friend extends his arm over and touches an object on the other side. "What's in there, what do you feel?" Now I can touch what I could not touch. He sticks his head over the wall; now it is my sense of smell that has been extended in range.

This raises two points. First, while it is possible that what my friend saw, felt, and smelled could be communicated to me by means of prosody—body and facial gesturing—this would most likely suffer in detail and clarity and thus *speed*, if the desired end result is to transmit the information accurately. This is usually the case with communication by any means, including deception through words or actions (the opossum who plays dead). For deception of any kind to achieve its desired result demands the clear outward expression of the internal abstraction; how truly this abstraction represents external reality is irrelevant. Only the clarity and accuracy with which the intent is conveyed is important.

A second point regarding the extension of the senses by means of spoken language concerns boundaries. The range of this extension is bounded by the range of the combination of the vocal and auditory elements of (this) communication. We can only yell so loudly and we can only hear from so far away. Thus, there are clear boundaries to this form of communication—and they seem rather constraining. But are they?

Let us say my friend is on a ladder now, looking over the same wall. I am just barely within earshot, and he yells to me what it is he sees. I turn and yell to another person just within ear shot, and so on and so forth. This chain of communication can allow someone far away to "see" with my friend's eyes as he peers over the wall. Now consider having cell phones.

There is no doubt this extension in the range of communication extends the range of the senses. There is also no doubt that early man learned this and used it to advantage, by sending messengers on foot and on horseback and by means of semaphores such as flags, smoke signals, and reflective surfaces added between nodes in this chain where word-to-word communication kept it moving. Here was a technique that conveyed information across great distances in segmented or nodal fashion, *not at all unlike the conduction of the action potential signal.*

But unlike the unfailing, unchanging action potential, the form of communication described above is limited. Although language increases the range of communication (and thus the theoretical range of the senses), it does so at the loss of both speed and accuracy. If you have noticed the distortion of information through gossip you will know what I mean. By the time the story cycles back, it has undergone a noticeable transformation and is distorted to the point of barely resembling the original at all. Although such distortion is often hilarious, in conditions where "pass the word" is important, it is not quite so funny when "one if by land, two if by sea" gets mixed up. The old adage that too many links makes the chain weak is very true in regards to spoken language, with "weak" here meaning deficient in detail, accuracy, and speed. Even if somehow the transmission of information is reliable and unchanging at each node from source to end in all chains of flow (pathway of communication), distortion of the overall signal will occur because of differences in the timing of reception on the part of the receiving elements. For appropriate impact, a given signal (message) almost always needs to reach many destinations rather than just one.

Let us look at information flow from a broader evolutionary context. Just as it took a long time for single cells to become animals, it has taken a long time for humans to evolve into a closely knit society, and the reason or reasons for this are basically the same. In the case of single cells, we saw in chapter 4 that cell grouping into multicellular animals required communication—*meaning*—between cells. This took a tremendous amount of time to develop. In even the most primitive cell colonies, the importance of simultaneity in signal reception is clear when we think of the combination of motor elements that must act in synchrony to perform successfully even the simplest of movements, such as the organized FAP of swimming in the lamprey. As the nervous system developed over evolution into its own society of cells, simultaneity of activation as a modular form underlying function was not only conserved, but increased in capability. As the need for more complicated movement increased, synchronous activation of widely differing muscle synergies became necessary. This was accomplished through both a coordinating timing signal from such sites as the inferior olivary nucleus, and the varied speed of conduction of fibers of different lengths assuring simultaneous arrival of the signal at target destinations across a wide range of distances.

At the evolutionary present, the most profound example of natural selection's conservation, embellishment, and incorporation of simultaneity of activation is the brain's solution to the problem of perceptual binding and its byproduct, cognition. Chapter 6, devoted solely to this issue, described the thalamocortical system as a close to isochronic (synchronized) sphere of function, binding in time the fractured elements of internal and external reality as represented by the neural activities of spatially disparate regions of the brain. According to this view, simultaneity of activation within this system results in perceptual unity: this book you feel in your hands, this voice that seems to be reading to you, the sense of the chair around you, all seem as one event, occurring now.

Imagine the problems with perceptual truth if simultaneous activation did not occur. Even within one sensory modality there would be trouble. If we could not bind in perceptual time what the tongue feels, the changing pressures the teeth feel, the sense of the roof of the mouth and inner cheeks, we would quickly destroy this multicomponent apparatus so important to us for the ingestion of food, among other things. If the timing of perception of these different tactile sensations were off even a little, the simple act of chewing one's dinner would result in a bitten tongue and lacerated cheeks.

Without simultaneity of activation the problems are compounded if there is an attempt to orchestrate more than one sense modality. We could never play a musical instrument, because what we hear and what we feel in our fingers would never match. We would be unable to enunciate words, or ride a bicycle. In short, without coordinated simultaneity of activation, the binding of activity of the various sensory systems into perceptual unity would be impossible, and without that the self would be left fragmented. Had evolution not solved the binding problem, we would not be discussing it now. Out of time, out of mind—literally.

Similarly, we can see that early in the formation of human society there was a need to solve the binding problem for information transfer. Messages were distorted by the fact that they were distributed at different speeds among different elements in the society and thus were not received simultaneously by everyone. Things change; what is important one day may not be the next, and so conflicting messages occur. The result is that consensus truth about the global—even local—state of affairs is neither complete nor stable.

Just as the evolution of the brain has solved the perceptual binding problem by its incorporation and use of simultaneity of activation, it is abstraction, a product of intrinsic brain activity, that has tightened the communicative fabric binding society together, in the sense of consensual truth of information. Beginning with communication through pictures and then the written word, abstract thinking has lead to a series of technological advances resulting in successively more accurate, detailed, and today virtually simultaneous communication between individuals separated by great distance. "One small step for a man, one giant leap for

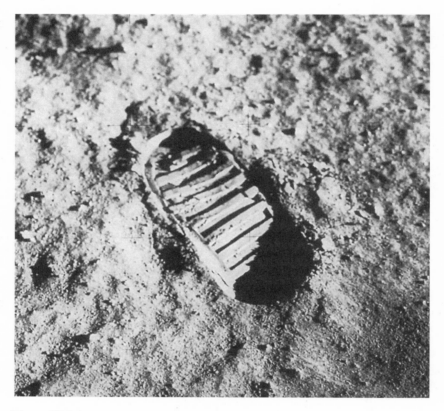

Figure 12.1
One small step for a man, one giant leap for mankind. Astronaut Edwin "Buzz" Aldrin's footprint in the lunar soil, made during the Apollo 11 mission in 1969, as part of an experiment to study the nature of lunar dust and the effects of pressure on the surface. (From website nssdc.gsfc.nasa.gov).

mankind" may sound banal, but as a riveting, historic moment it could be experienced by all of us on Earth at the same time, if not at the exact moment of its utterance (figure 12.1).

In the decade of the 1990s we have experienced the latest event in this series of communicative advancements: the World Wide Web. In all seriousness, it is fair to say that the Web represents a breakthrough in communication, perhaps second only in importance to the invention of written language itself. The first great advance altered the course of human civilization, and this second one may too. Just in its infancy, the

Web's presence has already profoundly reshaped the most developed societies, and will continue to do so in ways that are difficult to imagine now.

The Web: A Hub Perhaps, but a Collective Mind?

Other than the Web, let us consider what communication systems we have. A television signal can reach millions, as can newspapers, albeit a good deal more slowly. Neither is interactive. A given message or opinion is stated, we receive it, make our judgements, and there it stops. We may discuss it with friends, but we are not contributing in any real sense to that unidirectional flow of information. We may write to an editor, but this is in all likelihood just pebbles at an elephant, and worse still is that this interaction is painfully slow. Compared to a simple conversation at lunch, this is hardly interactive at all.

Telephone and certain forms of radio have the range and speed to allow virtually instantaneous transmission, but bidirectional communication flow quickly turns unidirectional when the number of users increases, even by a few. Any taxi driver will tell you that although one can *hear* the activity on a particular channel, as the number of users on that channel increases one can hardly get a word in edgewise. The frequency bandwidth is full and that happens, unfortunately, rather easily.

Telephones can connect you with just about anyone, anywhere, with negligible delay. But how many people can you interact with in this fashion? One could, in theory, fill an auditorium and address this crowd through an amplified speaker or conference phone, but if more than even two people respond, the result would be unintelligible noise. And so, again, bidirectional communication flow quickly becomes unidirectional as the number of users increases and interaction is reduced to listening or talking, but not both.

Much has changed since the time of Paul Revere, in that issues of detail, accuracy, range (serial range, anyway), and speed of communication no longer pose serious limitations to individual communication needs. The outer boundary of our capabilities becomes exposed only when we insist on bidirectional or interactive information flow that is virtually simultaneous over vast ranges and over vast numbers of sending and re-

http://www.

Figure 12.2
The World Wide Web.

ceiving parties. When we ask that communication flow as it does in the brain, the limitations of global information transfer are exposed.

But these limitations are disappearing. At least in theory, the Web is a nervous system-like structure in that its functioning seems to be solving, to a certain extent, society's binding problem (figure 12.2).

Already the Web provides communicative simultaneity of activation unlike anything the world has ever seen, allowing for a single person to post a message to thousands, hundreds of thousands, even millions of other people almost instantaneously. Moreover, interaction remains bidirectional at these numbers: any or all of these recipients may send their reply right back, the only delay being the amount of time it takes to frame one's thoughts and compose the reply. In other words, the delay is now for the most part no longer a technical one.

We see that the flow of information through the Web is similar to, and perhaps best analogized by, the flow of information between and among neurons, but will the Web demonstrate some sort of intrinsic embedding as well? If so, what will be embedded? We learned in chapters 3 and 8 that repetitious patterns of neural activity become recognized and incorporated into the nervous system's overall mode of operation (memories, FAPs, and the like), which at all times attempts to increase its computational efficiency while lowering its computational overhead. Intuitively, the increased speed and volume of information flow we see on the Web should feed well into this concept of embedding . . . but is this analogy real? And if so, will the results be beneficial?

If neurons beget mind, can the people—the *minds*—that represent each nodal point in the Web generate or become a collective mind? Can the Web support a consciousness of man, and if so, what on earth would *this* be like? On the surface, the Web and the brain are very different. The brain is *alive* and the Web is not. Can something nonbiological have a mind?

This last question is neither rhetorical nor limited to discussions concerning the Web. It is of potentially great importance to human society, and is one demanding thorough and concerted attention across many disciplines.

At first glance, the workings of the Web do appear to have some features in common with the workings of the brain, but even this pseudo-analogy falls apart rather quickly on closer scrutiny. At all times throughout this book, I have stressed a perspective of functional architecture, and viewed from this perspective the Web is awkward at best. In practice, the Web as it is would not be able to support a consciousness of many. For one, it is a very noisy system. Also, although very fast in tasks such as getting a message from here to there, it is not fast enough in its integrative parameters to support consciousness the way the nervous system does (which is still our best, if not only reference or standard). The nervous system, you should recall, increases its own efficiency through modularization of function (see Miklos 1993). The Web as it presently exists is not modular. Among all nervous systems it might be most closely analogized to that of a coelenterate—a hydra or jellyfish. And if there is indeed consciousness present in a jellyfish, it is not of a quality that would be capable of supporting, *en masse*, a collective mind. Ultimately what one needs is a subsystem to collect and another subsystem to distribute, with the simplest of interactions at the node where these two would come together.

The concept of a collective consciousness is not a new one. The outcome of an election is taken as a mandate of the people, representing a collective decision by the populace. For embedding, the benefits of interacting with a greater number of other minds and the experiences that each represent should be obvious, as the nervous system pays particular attention to new stimuli, and it embeds, for the most part, based on repetition. If one person in your life cautions, "Do not play with any black spider that has an hourglass on its belly," but then goes on to say, "You won't believe this, but I once saw a flying whale," you might remember the spider warning at about the time you are being bitten. On the other hand, if you were to hear this spider advice numerous times from friends, parents, teachers, and doctors, all warning you about what could happen to you if are bitten, you would probably steer clear of these spiders the first time you saw one. What sticks in the mind is the repetition, and the sense that this knowledge evolved from the repetitive swirling of the information between and across other minds before you.

But wait: collective knowledge and collective mind are not one and the same. Although there may be many definitions of collective mind, one we all may agree upon is that the elements comprising the whole combine in such a way that when confronted as a whole, a singular decision about what to do is formed and implemented. The decision that is formed may not and most likely will not be representative of each element's perspective or opinion, but rather is a consensus that serves to benefit the group overall. This is the same as the sacrifices made and benefits gained when single cells opt to socialize, leading eventually to multicellular organisms. This process culminates in the formation of a collective structure that assumes the role of the decision maker for the animal, namely the nervous system.

If we think seriously about what constitutes a collective mind, the Web is a promising candidate in terms of what it potentially might take to support a consciousness of many. It is certainly arguable that the Web has been created out of man's desire *to* create a collective mind.

Is the Web a nervous system composed of nervous systems, a mind composed of minds? Not yet, as I've said, not in the classical sense of collective mind. It is communicating, true, but it isn't thinking. A very similar form of global decision-making process is taking shape nonetheless, which is beginning—and will continue—to affect everyone, for better or worse.

"Eat Garbage: One Trillion Flies Cannot Be Wrong"

Should we believe that we should eat garbage? Is this logical? Is it *true*? This is the problem with numbers. The tyranny of the majority has always been an issue, and as most of us know, the document known as the U.S. Constitution was designed in part to protect the citizens from this threat. Nevertheless, if enough people want to have creationism taught alongside evolution in their schools as equally viable and unproven (and implicitly unprovable) theories, then so shall it be. The ability of the mass media to affect public opinion has been demonstrated many times, although, as we have said, mass media is not interactive like the Web or as responsive to one's ideas as the Web can be. So far, the public has been largely a passive receiver of information. However, for the first time, because of the incredible speed, range, and volume of communication the Web brings, public opinion could *truly* become public—with its inherent advantages and disadvantages.

Here is where the problem with numbers arises. The Web, precisely because of its speed and volume of information flow, may perpetuate the notion of weighting the value of ideas or beliefs based simply on the number of people reporting that they adhere to them. Not just tyranny of the majority, but of a biased, self-selected one at that! Two hundred thousand people contributing their opinions on an issue on the Web think this or that, ergo it *must* be true. Ultimately, this inertia of numbers develops a life of its own and determines whether we like or believe something or not, thus giving rise to the self-fulfilling prophecy. And this phenomenon will undoubtedly be accelerated by the machinations of the Web.

As individuals, we know that generalizations based on popular opinion are unreliable. But at the individual level, if you disagree with the inertia you will become an outsider and will therefore suffer the consequences of not being part of the group. Indeed, if anything one says can immediately be criticized by millions of people, it will quickly become very difficult to separate one's self from the beliefs and feelings of others. Under such pressures, homogenization of thinking will, of necessity, take place. As the Web becomes more intelligent, these machinations will have a strong influence on self-perception, and the very concept of self will become redefined. The concept of ideas as belonging to oneself will be diluted by the fact that any idea given to the Web will either gain acceptance, immediately being commonplace, or will be immediately rejected. This will whittle away our ability to discern individual identity, our possession of ideas—in essence, what forms the backbone of our beliefs in and of self. A homogenization of thought cannot help but occur, and this will, by further feeding the inertia of numbers, cycle against itself in a very implosive fashion.

Homogenization of thought will lead to the homogenization of society, a sobering prospect for the future. When traveling as a youngster, I always loved to see the richness of differences in cultures, beliefs, and viewpoints. Not so much today; for example, you find that children in

Asia or Europe or Africa all want the same consumer products, in part because they are bombarded by similar images from whatever media reaches them. The trend toward sameness is everywhere apparent, as everything, the good and the trite, is being copied—and in general, the trite is easier to copy than something that takes some thought. We are fast approaching a world culture of sameness not only in the external trappings, but also the character and values of societies. The strength of public media and its influence has made it almost impossible to buck this trend, and there is no reason to believe that the Web will not accelerate this process.

The true downside to homogenization is a decrease in variation, and variation is the key to survival. So the system becomes more brittle simply by the fact that options are reduced if everyone feels exactly the same about any event or given set of values. Against a background of sameness, vulnerabilities are more easily exposed—and more likely. We will look into this a bit later on.

A final point on the generation of a collective mind is that, as in evolution, trial and error must of necessity come into play. It might take as much time as it took nerve cells to make brains for us to learn how to implement such an extended awareness. If properly used this could be an extraordinary development. But as it is right now, the Web needs a serious overhaul in functional architecture to even hope to approach a collective event of the nature we have discussed.

Is it reasonable to consider the world order as being at all like that of the brain? Yes. What we observe is a similarity of order expressed at different levels, at *all* levels from cells to animals and from animals to societies. One wonders if this is perhaps a universal law. The way the system organizes itself may reflect, for example, its solution to the tyranny of the second law of thermodynamics, "order will decrease with time." There may be a deeper message here. One of the few ways in which local order can increase is through the generation of such things as a nervous system that employs *modularization of function*. If modularization is indeed a universal to combat disorder, such a geometric and architectural solution may have happened at other levels as well. Chances are high that the weak anthropomorphic principle, namely that we are here because the universal laws make it likely to the point of inevitability, is the underlying universal tendency, rather than the other way around (the strong anthropomorphic principle)—that a predetermined event in the distant past formed the universe in the way it did, so that we could "become."

Can I Stay Inside and Play?

The spawn of the technology behind the Web presents an ominous event if not properly modulated. If allowed to expand out of all control, it could become a danger, perhaps the most serious threat that society has ever encountered, eclipsing that of war, disease, famine, or drug problems. The event we should fear most is the possibility that as we develop better forms of communication with one another, we may cease to desire interaction with the external world. If one considers the problems for society of mind-altering drugs, then imagine if people could realize their dreams, any dreams, by means of virtual communication with other real or imaginary human beings. And not just via the visual system, but through *all* sensory systems. Keep in mind that the only reality that exists for us is already a virtual one—we are dreaming machines by nature! And so virtual reality can only feed on itself, with the risk that we can very easily bring about our own destruction.

If you consider how many hours a day people now watch TV, the amount of time that will be spent in virtual worlds can only be more because it is not just watching but *interacting*. You can play the music you are hearing. You can fly a plane, hunt an elephant, experience intimate sexual contact, virtually. Whatever you wish. The possibility of disrupting society is virtually boundless. It could be the ultimate intellectual dependency, because the true boundaries that reality defines would disappear. The hard facts of life could be seriously questioned. Here is the possibility of creating a totally hedonistic state, a decadent sybaritic society rushing headlong into self-destruction and oblivion. We all know that pleasure must be titrated; it must not be inhaled too deeply. Ideally, pleasure is not an end in itself but rather the means to an end. If we are approaching some form of collective consciousness, it may be a dangerously narcissistic one, one that could precipitate the unraveling of a society already undermined by the ominously anti-intellectual climate in which we live.

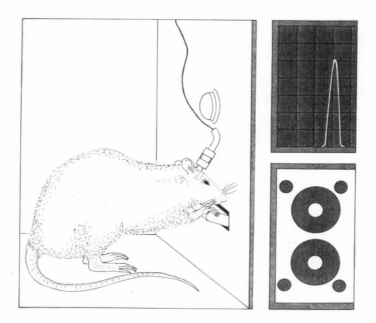

Figure 12.3
Uncontrolled self-stimulation. A Skinner-box apparatus is used to study the behavioral effects of brain reward. A metal electrode is implanted in the reward system of the rat, and the animal is allowed to trigger an electric stimulus to its brain by pressing the treadle. The curve on the oscilloscope screen indicates the delivery of the stimulus. If the stimulating electrode is implanted in the medial forebrain bundle of the hypothalamus, the rat will stimulate itself nearly continuously for days, neglecting food, water, and sleep. Other parts of reward system give rise to less dramatic effects. (From Routtenberg 1978.)

Brain research has known this for years. Place a stimulating electrode within a rat's medial forebrain bundle, the pleasure center of the brain. Now allow the rat free control to activate this area by pressing an electrically connected lever, and the rat will forego all food, sleep, and water to stay in a state of constant bliss. And it will stay there until it is dead (figure 12.3). Humans will lethally titrate cocaine intake in the same way. Virtual reality will be a lever in this regard, possibly greater and more powerfully addicting than any we have seen yet. Life itself is not a dream; it is about physical survival and continuation. Virtual reality will not fill the need.

Hopefully, the wisdom of human nature will ultimately recognize this virtual realm as nonreal: that somehow the evolutionary event would by some quirk have known that something like this was possible. That somehow our brains evolved not to allow us to act out our REM-driven dreams lest we hurt ourselves. More realistically, one can hope that evolution might resolve the problem much as it resolves great natural catastrophes, through variation and selection. A small subset of people may be found who say, "Don't give me any of that two-dimensional sex, I want the real thing." The culling of society through natural selection might produce a different, more thoughtful human being. It may be all that we can hope for.

Mindness Is not Necessarily a Property of Biology Alone

Whether the Web is alive in a biological sense or not is probably irrelevant. If we consider each opinion, belief, or message from an individual as a stimulus, then the Web acts much as consciousness does. It makes quick, yea or nay consensus decisions about incoming stimuli and generates a solution; there simply is no time for anything else.

Discussions of this nature suggest an obvious, ultimate question: Is mindness a property that can reside only within the realm of the biological, or living flesh and blood?

Let us think for a moment about the case of flight. If it were the thirteenth or fourteenth century, we might conclude that flight is a property of biology, perhaps exclusively so from the fact that the only objects that are heavier than air and that can fly are living creatures. By contrast, every person living at the end of the twentieth century now knows that flying is not a property exclusive to biology. Similarly, one may wonder if mindness is exclusively a biological property. Computers as we know them today do not seem ready to have a mind, but that may be due more to limitations in our choice of design architecture than to any theoretical constraint on artificially created mindness. In the case of flight, specialized skin, cuticle tissue, and feathers have all proven their worth as materials in the composite that conquers gravity—as have plastic, dead wood, and various metals. It is not just the materials, but the design that defines feasibility here.

So is "mind" a property of biology alone, or is it actually a physical property that may in theory be supported by some nonbiological architecture? Put another way, is there any serious reason to believe that biology is separate from physics? The scientific knowledge gathered over the last hundred years or so suggests that biology, in all its amazing complexity, is no different from anything else that obeys the laws of physics. Thus it should be possible for consciousness to be implemented by a physical organism, which in our case happens to be what we call a biological system.

The question that people generally ask is somewhat different: whether devices of an other than biological nature are capable of supporting consciousness, qualia, memory, and awareness, that which we consider to be the serious properties of nervous system function. That is, would a computer ever really be able to think?

The easy answer is yes, we think they can and will. But the more relevant question is: What would the physical system have to be like or look like before it can do the same as the brain? Or, perhaps, as some still feel, is there something spooky or otherwise indefinable, not knowable, in brain, that which in philosophy has been called the "hard problem"? It seems to me that the issue is most likely one of physical degrees of freedom of functional architecture, rather than the aliveness of biology versus the deadness of physics.

Having been a vertebrate physiologist all my life, with some forays into the invertebrate world, I have presented in this book an image of consciousness that is embodied by a particular type of neural network or circuit. But I must tell you one of the most alarming experiences I've had in pondering brain function. This was the realization, from discussions with Roger Hanlin at the Marine Biological Laboratory at Woods Hole, that the octopus is capable of truly extraordinary feats of intelligence. I have read of experiments in octopus by J. Z. Young (1989), where these invertebrates have solved problems as complicated as opening a jar to remove a crab kept inside. Operating with nothing but the visual image and olfactory clues indicating the presence of the crab inside and the tactile manipulation of the jar, the creature finally found that the top could be opened by applying force. And after having done so, when presented again with the same problem, the animal was immediately capable of

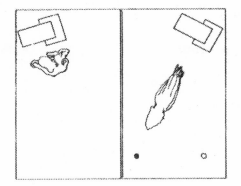

Figure 12.4
The remarkable octopus. Schematic of the experimental apparatus and protocol. An *Octopus vulgaris* is shown (*right*) attacking a ball (the dark one) and acting as a demonstrator for the other animal (observer, *left*), which is standing outside of its home and watching its conspecific during the whole session through a transparent wall. Each tank had an independent supply of running water. Octopi were allowed to visually interact for 2 hours before the start of the observational phase. Mean duration of the trials, which depended on the demonstrator's performances, was 40 seconds, and the period between trials was 5 minutes. (From Fiorito and Scotto, 1992, figure 1, p. 545.)

opening the top and fetching the crab out. Astoundingly, this event could be learned with a single trial. More to the point, however, and most remarkable is the report that octopi may learn from observing other octopi at work (figure 12.4). The alarming fact here is that the organization of the nervous system of this animal is *totally* different from the organization we have learned is capable of supporting this type of activity in the vertebrate brain (see Miklos 1993). If we are faced with the sobering fact that there are two possible solutions to the "intelligence" problem, then there may well be a large number of possible architectures that could provide the basis of what we consider necessary for cognition and qualia. On the other hand, it may be that although we have observed great intelligence in animals such as the octopus or *Sepia*, these creatures might not in fact have anything like qualia. My position, though, is that the simplest assumption from what we see is that their behavior supports subjectivity. Given the principle of parsimony, the onus of proof lies with those who believe that these animals are devoid of qualia.

But is there something in principle quite different from the types of embodiments that we have in modern day computers and in the nervous system itself? That is a very serious and important question to ask. One may consider, as did Alan Turing (Turing 1947; Millican and Clark 1996), whether it is in principle possible to make a universal machine out of a digital type of device if the appropriate algorithms are implemented. Can algorithmic computation ever be sufficiently extensive, fast, and concise enough to implement the totality of properties that a 14-watt entity such as our brain can implement with 1.5 kilograms of mass? And what do we make of the intelligence of an ant that as a robot demonstrates incredible computational agility with mere milligrams of neuronal mass, a brain with less mass than a single microchip? The fundamental issue is that brains are nothing like digital computers; they operate as analog devices and thus utilize physics directly in their measurements, as opposed to the abstracted measures of zeros and ones that are cleansed of the elements that generated them. Is the computation of digital physical computers truly comparable to that performed by analog devices? It has been stated that for a digital computer to be able to support the equivalent computational properties (capabilities) of the brain, the mass required might be many orders of magnitude larger and the power supply equally as large.

There is another argument to consider in terms of the differences between brains and computers. Warren McCulloch wondered long ago how it was that reliability could arise from nonreliable systems (McCulloch 1965). The reader should know by now how unreliable nerve cells are as computational entities. First of all, they have intrinsic activity, and thus as conveyors and relayers of information may be extremely noisy. McCulloch's answer was rather intriguing: he felt that reliability could be attained if neurons were organized in parallel so that the ultimate message was the sum of activity of the neurons acting simultaneously. He further explained that a system where the elements were unreliable to the point that their unreliabilities were sufficiently different from one another would in principle be far *more* reliable than a system made out of totally reliable parts. Here, a reliable system is one with unreliability in each element as low as possible but still present.

This may sound almost paradoxical, but in what is considered a reliable system, the elements are reliable to about the same extent. And even if this reliability is 99.99 percent, the problem is that the elements are also all the same in their unreliability, *meaning that what is unreliable is common to all the elements.* It therefore becomes an issue of probabilities. In such reliable or redundant systems then, whatever tiny problem or unreliability they do have will *add up.* In nonreliable systems, however, the elements are *not* redundant and are therefore slightly different in their unreliability. Because they are all slightly different in their unreliability, there will never be the possibility of this unreliability adding up! These unreliable systems are therefore far more reliable than reliable systems. The flip side of this is that in a system with elements of differing unreliabilities, what they have in common are the reliable aspects! This is fundamental. It means that for an instrument to be totally reliable it must ultimately be made up of unreliable—varied—parts!

Herein lies precisely the fragility of society we may experience from the homogenizing effect of the Web on our thoughts, ideas, beliefs, and the like. As variation decreases, things become increasingly redundant and unreliability becomes the prevailing commonality across the elements—and in the case of society, *we* are the elements.

Returning to the implementation of consciousness and so-called artificial (nonbiological) intelligence, it is possible that until we can understand the issue of unreliability and the probabilistic nature of computation in analog systems, we will not be able to generate the required architecture. With the proper functional architecture we could probably generate consciousness in a very large set of nonbiological entities.

The second issue is one of knowledge of self. Suppose a potential embodiment of consciousness is allowed the necessary freedom to explore and internalize the external world such that an image of self, however primitive it may be, is implemented. While this embodiment may measure external reality, the possibility of having an entity that is aware in the sense we mean most probably will not ever arise. We know that this is fundamental in the functioning of the nervous system. It can be seen in individuals who are given inverted prisms that make the world appear visually upside down. These individuals will learn to use the visual image as if right side-up *only* if allowed to interact in a motor sense with that image. They must move within it to adjust. Ultimately we see that *the architecture capable of generating cognition must relate to the motricity upon which such cognition was developed.* To be conscious, computers must move and manipulate—they must be robots. Without such self-reference, the issue of syntax versus semantics will always come up (see the Chinese room paradigm; Searle 1992) as consciousness is ultimately simply context-dependent.

When the architectures for generating cognition are finally realized, we may have thinking/feeling machines. However, our ability to design and build them may not ultimately be that useful in understanding brain function, in the same way that understanding airplanes may not tell us all about how the physiology of bats or birds enables them to fly.

References

Abbott, L. F., Rolls, E. T., and Tovee, M. J. (1996). Representational capacity of face coding in monkeys. *Cereb. Cortex.* 6: 498–505.

Abel, T., and Kandel, E. (1998). Positive and negative regulatory mechanisms that mediate long-term memory storage. *Brain Res. Rev.* 26: 360–378.

Aboitiz, F., and Garcia, R. (1997a). The anatomy of language revisited. *Biol. Res.* 30: 171–183.

Aboitiz, F., and Garcia, R. (1997b). The evolutionary origin of the language areas in the human brain. A neuroanatomical perspective. *Brain Res. Rev.* 25: 381–396.

Adrianov, O. S. (1996). Cerebral interrelationships of cognitive and emotional activity: Pathways and mechanisms. *Neurosci. Behav. Physiol.* 26: 329–339.

Ali, M. A., ed. (1984). *Photoreception and Vision in Invertebrates.* New York: Plenum.

Archer, S. M., Helveston, E. M., Miller, K. K., and Ellis, F. D. (1986). Stereopsis in normal infants and infants with congenital esotropia. *Am. J. Ophthalmol.* 101: 591–596.

Armstrong, D. L., Turin, L., and Warner, A. E. (1983). Muscle activity and the loss of electrical coupling between striated muscle cells in *Xenopus* embryos. *J. Neurosci.* 3: 1414–1421.

Arnold, A. P. (1975a). The effects of castration on song development in zebra finches (*Poephila guttata*). *J. Exp. Zool.* 191: 261–278.

Arnold, A. P. (1975b). The effects of castration and androgen replacement on song, courtship, and aggression in zebra finches (*Poephila guttata*). *J. Exp. Zool.* 191:309–326.

Arshavsky, Y. I., Deliagina, T. G., and Orlovsky, G. N. (1997). Pattern generation. *Curr. Opin. Neurobiol.* 7: 781–789.

Bailey, C. H., Bartsch, D., and Kandel, E. R. (1996). Toward a molecular definition of long-term memory storage. *Proc. Natl. Acad. Sci. USA.* 93: 13445–13452.

Baker, T. C., Cosse, A. A., and Todd, J. L. (1998). Behavioral antagonism in the moth *Helicoverpa zea* in response to pheromone blends of three sympatric heliothine moth species is explained by one type of antennal neuron. *Ann. NY Acad. Sci.* 855: 511–513.

Banks, W. P. (1996). How much work can a quale do? *Conscious Cogn.* 5: 368–380.

Bard P. (1928). A diencephalic mechanism for the expression of rage with special reference to the sympathetic nervous system. *Amer. J. Physiol.* 84: 490–515.

Bateson, P. P. G. (1966). The characteristics and context of imprinting. *Biological Review* 41: 177–220.

Batueva, I. V. (1987). Efficiency of electrical transmission in reticulo-motoneuronal synapses of lamprey spinal cord. *Exp. Brain Res.* 69: 131–139.

Batueva, I. V., and Shapovalov, A. I. (1977). Electrotonic and chemical EPSPs in lamprey motor neurons following stimulation of the descending tract and posterior root afferents. *Neirofiziologiia* 9: 512–517. [Article in Russian]

Bear, M. F., Conners, B. W., and Paradiso, M. A. (1996). *Neuroscience: Exploring the Brain.* Baltimore: Williams and Wilkins.

Beeckmans, K., and Michiels, K. (1996). Personality, emotions and the temporolimbic system: A neuropsychological approach. *Acta Neurol. Belg.* 96: 35–42.

Bekoff, A., Stein, P. S. G., and Hamburger, V. (1975). Co-ordinated motor output in the hindlimb of the 7-day chick embryo. *Proc. Natl. Acad. Sci. USA* 72: 1245–1248.

Benini, A. (1998). Pain as a biological phenomenon of consciousness. *Schweiz Rundsch Med. Prax.* 87: 224–228.

Benke, T., Bosch, S., and Andree, B. (1998). A study of emotional processing in Parkinson's disease. *Brain Cogn.* 38: 36–52.

Bennett, M. V. L. (1971). Electric organs. In: *Fish Physiology,* W. S. Hoar, D. J. Randall, eds. New York: Academic Press, pp. 347–391.

Bennett, M. V. L. (1997). Gap junctions as electrical synapses. *J. Neurocytol.* 26: 349–366.

Bennett, M. V. L. (2000). Electrical synapses, a personal perspective (or history). *Brain Res. Brain Res. Rev.* 32: 16–28.

Bennett, M. V. L, and Pappas, G. D. (1983). The electromotor system of the stargazer: A model for integrative actions at electrotonic synapses. *J. Neurosci.* 3: 748–761.

Bennett, M. V. L, Sandri, C., and Akert, K. (1989). Fine structure of the tuberous electroreceptor of the high-frequency electric fish, *Sternarchus albifrons* (gymnotiformes). *J. Neurocytol.* 18: 265–283.

Berardelli, A. (1995). Symptomatic or secondary basal ganglia diseases and tardive dyskinesias. *Curr. Opin. Neurol.* 8: 320–322.

Berardelli, A., Rothwell, J. C., Hallett, M., Thompson, P. D., Manfredi, M., and Marsden, C. D. (1998). The pathophysiology of primary dystonia. *Brain* 121: 1195–1212.

Bernard, J. F., Bester, H., and Besson, J. M. (1996). Involvement of the spino-parabrachio-amygdaloid and -hypothalamic pathways in the autonomic and affective emotional aspects of pain. *Prog. Brain Res.* 107: 243–255.

Bernstein, N. A. (1967). *The Coordination and Regulation of Movements.* Oxford: Pergamon Press.

Bevans, C. G., Kordel, M., Rhee, S. K., Harris, A. L. (1998). Isoform composition of connexin channels determines selectivity among second messengers and uncharged molecules. *J. Biol. Chem.* 273: 2808–16.

Bizzi, E., Saltiel, P., and Tresch, M. (1998). Modular organization of motor behavior. *Z. Naturforsch.* 53: 510–517.

Blackshaw, S. E., and Warner, A. E. (1976). Low resistance junctions between mesoderm cells during development of trunk muscles. *J. Physiol. (Lond.)* 255: 209–230.

Bleasel, A. F., and Pettigrew A. G. (1992). Development and properties of spontaneous oscillations of the membrane potential in inferior olivary neurons in the rat. *Brain Res. De. Brain Res.* 65: 43–50.

Block, N. (1995). The Mind as the software of the brain. In *An Invitation to Cognitive Science,* ed. D. Osheron, L. Gleitman, S. Kosslyn, E. Smith and S. Steinberg, ed. Cambridge: MIT Press.

Braddick, O. (1996). Binocularity in infancy. *Eye.* 10: 182–188.

Broca, P. (1861). *Memoire sur le cerveau de l'homme.* Paris: Reinwald.

Brooks, V. B. (1983) Motor control: How posture and movements are governed. *Phys. Ther.* 63: 664–673.

Brown, G. (1911). The intrinsic factors in the act of progression in the mammal. *Proc. Roy. Soc. Lond.* B. 84: 308–319.

Brown, G. (1914). On the nature of the fundamental activity of nervous centers *J. Physiol.* 48: 18–46.

Brown, G. (1915). On the activities of the central nervous system; together with an analysis of the conditioning of rhythmic activity in progression and a theory of the evolution of the nervous system. *J. Physiol.* 49: 18–46.

Brown, K. S. (1983). Evolution and development of the dentition. *Birth Defects Orig. Artic. Ser.* 19: 29–66.

Brown, S., and Schafer, A. (1888). An investigation into the functions of the occipital and temporal lobes of the monkey's brain. *Phil. Trans. R. Soc. London B. Biol. Sci.* 179: 303–327.

Camperi, M., and Wang, X. J. (1998). A model of visuospatial working memory in prefrontal cortex: Recurrent network and cellular bistability. *J. Comput. Neurosci.* 5: 383–405.

Casey, K. L. (1999). Forebrain mechanisms of nociception and pain: Analysis through imaging. *Proc. Natl. Acad. Sci. USA.* 96: 7668–7674.

Chalmers, D. J. (1995). Facing up to the problem of consciousness. *J. Consciousness Studies* 2: 200–219.

Chalmers, D. J. (1996). *The Conscious Mind: In Search of a Fundamental Theory.* New York: Oxford University Press.

Chalmers, D. J. (1997). Moving forward on the problem of consciousness. *J. Consciousness Studies* 4: 3–46.

Chang, Q., Pereda, A., Pinter, M. J., and Balice-Gordon R. J. (2000). Nerve injury induces gap junctional coupling among axotomized adult motor neurons. *J. Neurosci.* 20: 674–684.

Changeux, J. P. (1996) *The Neuronal Man.* Princeton: Princeton University Press.

Changeux, J. P. and Deheane, S. (2000). Hierarchical modeling of cognitive functions: From synaptic transmission to the Tower of London. *Int. J. Psychol. Physiol.* 35: 179–187.

Charney, D. S., and Deutch, A. (1996). A functional neuroanatomy of anxiety and fear: Implications for the pathophysiology and treatment of anxiety disorders. *Crit. Rev. Neurobiol.* 10: 419–446.

Chelazzi, L., Duncan, J., Miller, E. K., and Desimone, R. (1998). Responses of neurons in inferior temporal cortex during memory-guided visual search. *J. Neurophysiol.* 80: 2918–2940.

Chomsky, N. (1964). The development of grammar in child language: Formal discussion. *Monogr. Soc. Res. Child Dev.* 29: 35–39.

Chomsky, N. (1967). Recent contributions to the theory of innate ideas. *Synthese* 17: 2–11.

Chomsky, N. (1968) *Language and Mind.* New York: Harcourt, Brace and World.

Chomsky, N. (1972). *Language and Mind.* New York: Harcourt, Brace and World.

Chomsky, N. (1980). Rules and representations. *Behav. and Brain Sci.* 3: 1–16.

Chomsky, N. (1986). Analytic study of the Tadoma method: Language abilities of three deaf-blind subjects. *J. Speech Hear. Res.* 29: 332–347.

Christensen, B. N. (1976). Morphological correlates of synaptic transmission in lamprey spinal cord. *J. Neurophysiol.* 39: 197–212.

Churchland, P. M. and Churchland, P. S. (1998). Recent work on consciousness: Philosophical, theoretical, and empirical. In *On the Contrary: Critical Essays, 1987–1997.* Cambridge: MIT Press.

Churchland, P. S. (1986). *Neurophilosophy: Toward a Unified Understanding of the Mind-Brain.* Cambridge: MIT Press.

Clayton, D. F. (1997). Role of gene regulation in song circuit development and song learning. *J. Neurobiol.* 33: 549–571.

Cloney, R. A. (1982). Ascidian larvae and the events of metamorphosis. *Am. Zool.* 22: 817–826.

Coffey, B. J., Miguel, E. C., Savage, C. R., Rauch, S. L. (1994). Tourette's disorder and related problems: A review and update. *Harv. Rev. Psychiatry.* 2: 121–132.

Cohen, A. (1987). Effects of oscillator frequency on phase-locking in the lamprey central pattern generator. *J. Neurosci. Methods.* 21: 113–125.

Colcher, A., and Simuni, T. (1999). Clinical manifestations of Parkinson's disease. *Med. Clin. North Am.* 83: 327–347.

Cole, J. A., Mohan, S., and Dow, C. (eds.) (1992). *Prokaryotic Structure and Function: A New Perspective.* Society for General Microbiology Symposium, no. 47. Cambridge: Cambridge University Press.

Cook, P. M., Prusky, G., and Ramoa, A. S. (1999). The role of spontaneous retinal activity before eye opening in the maturation of form and function in the retinogeniculate pathway of the ferret. *Vis. Neurosci.* 16: 491–501.

Cope, F. W. (1976). Derivation of the Weber-Fechner law and the Loewenstein equation as the steady-state response of an Elovich solid state biological system. *Bull. Math. Biol.* 38: 111–118.

Crick, F. C. H. (1991). *The Astonishing Hypothesis: The Scientific Search for the Soul.* New York: Touchstone Books.

Crick, F. C. H., and Koch C. (1990). Towards a neurological theory of consciousness. *Semin. Neurosci.* 2: 263–275.

Crook, J. H. (1983). On attributing consciousness to animals. *Nature* 303: 11–14.

Cropper, E. C., and Weiss, K. R. (1996). Synaptic mechanisms in invertebrate pattern generation. *Curr. Opin. Neurobiol.* 6: 833–841.

Damasio, A. (1994). *Descartes' Error.* New York: Putnam.

Damasio, A. (1999). *The Feeling of What Happens.* New York: Harcourt Brace and Co.

Damasio, A. R., Damasio, H., and Van Hoesen, G. W. (1982). Prosopagnosia: Anatomic basis and behavioral mechanisms. Neurology. 32: 331–341.

D'arcy W. Thompson. (1992). *On growth and form.* Cambridge, UK: Cambridge University Press.

Darwin, C. (1872). *The Expression of Emotions in Man and Animals*. London: John Murray, Publisher.

Davis, L. (1982). What is it like to be an agent? *Erkenntnis* 18: 195–213.

Davis, M. (1998). Anatomic and physiologic substrates of emotion in an animal model. *J. Clin. Neurophysiol.* 15: 378–387.

Davis, P. J., Zhang, S. P., Winkworth, A., and Bandler, R. (1996). Neural control of vocalization: Respiratory and emotional influences. *J. Voice.* 10: 23–38.

DeHaan, R. L., and Sachs, H. G. (1972). Cell coupling in developing systems: The heart-cell paradigm. *Curr. Top. Dev. Biol.* 7: 193–228.

Deiters O. (1865). In M. Schultze, ed. *Unter schungen über Gehim und Rückenmark des Menschen und der Sängethiere*. Braunschweig Wieweg.

Deliagina, T. G., Orlovsky, G. N., and Pavlova, G. A. (1983). The capacity for generation of rhythmic oscillations is distributed in the lumbosacral spinal cord of the cat. *Exp. Brain Res.* 53: 81–90.

Dennet, D. C. (1993). *Consciousness Explained*. New York: Penguin.

De Renzi E. de Pellegrino G. (1998). Prosopagnosia and alexia without object agnosia. *Cortex* 34: 403–15.

Devinsky, O., Morrell, M. J., and Vogt, B. A. (1995). Contributions of anterior cingulate cortex to behaviour. *Brain*. 118: 279–306.

DeVoogd, T. J. (1991). Endocrine modulation of the development and adult function of the avian song system. *Psychoneuroendocrinology*.16: 41–66.

DeVoogd, T. J., and Nottebohm, F. (1981). Sex differences in dendritic morphology of a song control nucleus in the canary: A quantitative Golgi study. *J. Comp. Neurol.* 196: 309–316.

Dewsbury, D. A., and Rethlingshafer, D. A. (1973). *Comparative psychology: A modern survey*. New York: McGraw-Hill, pp. 125–127.

De Zeeuw, C. I., Lang, E. J., Sugihara, I., Ruigrok, T. J., Eisenman, L. M., Mugnaini, E., and Llinás, R. (1996). Morphological correlates of bilateral synchrony in the rat cerebellar cortex. *Neurosci.* 16: 3412–3426.

Doty, R. L. (1986). Odor-guided behavior in mammals. *Experientia.* 42: 257–271.

Doupe, A. J. (1993). A neural circuit specialized for vocal learning. *Curr. Opin. Neurobiol.* 3: 104–111.

Doupe, A. J., and Konishi, M. (1991). Song-selective auditory circuits in the vocal control system of the zebra finch. *Proc. Natl. Acad. Sci. USA* 88: 11339–11343.

Doupe, A. J., and Kuhl, P. K. (1999). Birdsong and human speech: Common themes and mechanisms. *Annu. Rev. Neurosci.* 22: 567–631.

Downer J. C. D. (1961). Changes in the visual gnostic function and emotional behavior following unilateral temporal lobe damage in the "split-brain" monkey. *Nature* 191: 50–51.

Duchesne de Boulogne, G.-B. (1862). [Mecanisme de la Physionomie Humaine]. *The Mechanism of Human Facial Expression*. Edited and translated by R. A. Cuthbertson, 1990. Cambridge UK: Cambridge University Press.

Dyer, A. B., and Gottlieb, G. (1990). Auditory basis of maternal attachment in ducklings (*Anas platyrhynchos*) under simulated naturalistic imprinting conditions. *J. Comp. Psychol.* 104: 190–194.

Dyer, A. B., Lickliter, R., and Gottlieb, G. (1989). Maternal and peer imprinting in mallard ducklings under experimentally simulated natural social conditions. *Dev. Psychobiol.* 22: 463–475.

Eccles, J. C., Llinás, R., and Sasaki, K. (1966). The excitatory synaptic action of climbing fibres on the Purkinje cells of the cerebellum. *J. Physiol.* 182: 268–296.

Eckhorn, R., Bauer, R., Jordan, W., Brosch, M., Kruse, W., Munk, M., and Reitbock, H. J. (1988). Coherent oscillations: A mechanism of feature linking in the visual cortex? *Biol. Cybern.* 60: 121–130.

Edelman, G. M. (1992). *Bright Air, Brilliant Fire: On the Matter of the Mind*. New York: Basic Books.

Edelman, G. M. (1993). Neural Darwinism: Selection and reentrant signaling in higher brain function. *Neuron.* 10: 115–125.

Eglen, S. J. (1999). The role of retinal waves and synaptic normalization in retinogeniculate development. *Philos. Trans. R. Soc. Lond. B Biol. Sci.* 354: 497–506.

Elsen F. P., and Ramirez, J. M. (1998). Calcium currents of rhythmic neurons recorded in the isolated respiratory network of neonatal mice. *J. Neurosci.* 18: 10652–10662

Erecinska, M., and Silver, I. A. (1994). Ions and energy in the mammalian brain. *Prog. Neurobiol.* 43: 37–71.

Estevez-Gonzalez, A., Garcia-Sanchez, C., and Barraquer-Bordas, L. (1997). Memory and learning: "experience" and "skill" of the brain. *Rev. Neurol.* 25: 1976–1988. [Article in Spanish]

Fatt, P., and Katz, B. (1952). Spontaneous subthreshold activity at motor nerve endings. *J. Physiol. (Lond.)* 117: 109–128.

Feinberg, T. E. (1997). The irreducible perspectives of consciousness. *Semin. Neurol.* 17: 85–93.

Feldman, J. L., Smith, J. C., Ellenberger H. H., Connelly C. A., Liu G., Greer J. J., Lindsay, A. D., and Otto, M. R. (1990). Neurogenesis of respiratory rhythm and pattern-emerging concepts. *Am. J. Physiol.* 259: 879–886.

Ferguson, G., Messenger, J., and Budelmann, B. (1994). Gravity and light influence the countershading reflexes of the cuttlefish *Sepia officinalis*. *J. Exp. Biol.* 191: 247–256.

Fernandez de Molina, A. (1991). El cambio cerebral en la emoción. *Anales Real Acad. Nac. Medicina Madrid,* 1–109.

Fernandez de Molina, A., and Husperger R. W. (1959). Central representation of affective reactions in forebrain and brainstem: Electrical stimulation of amygdala, stria terminalis, and adjacent structures. *J. Physiol.* 145: 251–265.

Fernandez de Molina, A., and Husperger R. W. (1962). Organization of the subcortical system governing defence and flight reactions in the cat. *J. Physiol.* 160: 200–213.

Feynman R. P., and Hibbs, A. R. (1965). Quantum mechanics and path integrals New York: McGraw-Hill.

Fiorito, G., Scotto, P. (1992). Observational learning in *Octopus vulgaris*. *Science.* 256: 545–547.

Furshpan, E. J., and Potter, D. D. (1959). Transmission of giant motor synapses of the cray fish. *J. Physiol.* 145: 289–325.

Fuster, J. M. (1998). Distributed memory for both short and long term. *Neurobiol. Learn. Mem.* 70: 268–274.

Fuster, J. M., and Uyeda, A. A. (1971). Reactivity of limbic neurons of the monkey to appetitive and aversive signals. *EEG Clin. Neurophys.* 30: 281–293.

Gahr, M., and Garcia-Segura, L. M. (1996). Testosterone-dependent increase of gap-junctions in HVC neurons of adult female canaries. *Brain Res.* 712: 69–73.

Galambos, R., Makeig, S., and Talmachoff, P. J. (1981). A 40-Hz auditory potential recorded from the human scalp. *Proc. Natl. Acad. Sci.* 78: 2643–2547.

Ganger, J., and Stromswold, K. (1998). Innateness, evolution, and genetics of language. *Hum. Biol.* 70: 199–213.

Gannon, P. J., Holloway, R. L., Broadfield, D. C., and Braun, A. R. (1998). Asymmetry of chimpanzee planum temporale: Humanlike pattern of Wernicke's brain language area homolog. *Science.* 279: 220–222.

Gerhardstein, P., Adler, S. A., and Rovee-Collier, C. (2000). A dissociation in infants' memory for stimulus size: Evidence for the early development of multiple memory systems. *Dev. Psychobiol.* 36: 123–135.

Geschwind, N. (1965). The disconnexion syndrome in animals and man. *Brain* 88: 237–294.

Glassman, R. B. (1999). A working memory "theory of relativity": Elasticity in temporal, spatial, and modality dimensions conserves item capacity in radial maze, verbal tasks, and other cognition. *Brain Res. Bull.* 48: 475–489.

Goldman-Rakic, P. S. (1987). Circuitry of primate prefrontal cortex and regulation of behavior by representational memory. In F. Plum, V. B. Mountcastle (eds).

Handbook of Physiology. Sect. 1, *The Nervous System.* Vol. 5, *Higher Functions of the Brain,* Part 1, pp. 373–417. Bethesda, MD: Am. Physiol. Society.

Goldman-Rakic, P. S. (1992). Working memory and the mind. *Sci. Am.* 267: 111–117.

Goldman-Rakic, P. S. (1996). Memory: Recording experience in cells and circuits: Diversity in memory research. *Proc. Natl. Acad. Sci. USA* 93: 13435–13437.

Goldman-Rakic, P. S., Funahashi, S., and Bruce, C. J. (1990). Neocortical memory circuits. *Cold Spring Harb. Symp. Quant. Biol.* 55: 1025–1038.

Goller, F., and Larsen, O. N. (1997a). A new mechanism of sound generation in songbirds. *Proc. Natl. Acad. Sci. USA* 94: 14787–14791.

Goller, F., and Larsen, O. N. (1997b). In situ biomechanics of the syrinx and sound generation in pigeons. *J. Exp. Biol.* 200: 2165–2176.

Goller, F., and Suthers, R. A. (1996a). Role of syringeal muscles in controlling the phonology of bird song. *J. Neurophysiol.* 76: 287–300.

Goller, F., and Suthers, R. A. (1996b). Role of syringeal muscles in gating airflow and sound production in singing brown thrashers. *J. Neurophysiol.* 75: 867–876.

Goodman, D., and Kelso, J. A. (1983). Exploring the functional significance of physiological tremor: A biospectroscopic approach. *Exp. Brain Res.* 49: 419–431.

Gordon, N. Speech, language, and the cerebellum. 1996. *Eur. J. Disord. Commun.* 31: 359–367.

Gould, E., Reeves, A. J., Graziano, M. S. A., and Gross, C. G. (1999). Neurogenesis in the neocortex of adult primates. *Science* 286: 548–552.

Gould, J. L. (1976). The Dance-language controversy. The quarterly review of biology. *Q. Rev. Biol.* 51: 211–244.

Gould, J. L. (1990). Honey bee cognition. *Cognition.* 37: 83–103.

Gould, J. L., and Gould, C. G. (1989). *Life at the Edge. Readings from Scientific American Magazine.* New York: W.H. Freeman and Co.

Gould, S. J. (199?) Lecture entitled: Unity of Organic Design: From Goethe and Geoffroy Chaucer to Homology of Homeotic Complexes in Arthropods and Vertebrates, presented at New York University in honor of Homer Smith.

Gray, C. M., Konig, P. L., Engel, A. K., and Singer, W. (1989). Oscillatory responses in cat visual cortex exhibit inter-columnar synchronization which reflects global stimulus properties. *Nature* 338: 334–337.

Gray, C. M., and Singer, W. (1989). Stimulus-specific neuronal oscillations in orientation columns of cat visual cortex. *Proc. Nat. Acad. Sci. USA.* 86: 1698–1702.

Graybiel, A. M. (1995). Building action repertories: Memory and learning functions of the basal ganglion. *Curr. Opin. Neurobiol.* 5: 733–741.

Greene, P. H. (1972). Problems of organization of motor systems. In R. Rosen and F. M. Snell (eds.) *Progress in Theoretical Biology,* Vol. 2. New York: Academic, pp. 303–338.

Greene, P. H. (1982). Why is it easy to control your arms? *J. Motor Behav.* 14: 260–286.

Greenfield, P. M., and Savage-Rumbaugh, E. S. (1993). Comparing communicative competence in child and chimp: The pragmatics of repetition. *J. Child. Lang.* 20: 1–26.

Greenfield, S. A. (1995). *Journey to the Centers of the Mind.* New York: W. H. Freeman.

Gregory, R. L. (1988). Questions of quanta and qualia: Does sensation make sense of matter—or does matter make sense of sensation? Part 1. *Perception* 17: 699–702.

Gregory, R. L. (1989). Questions of quanta and qualia: Does sensation make sense of matter—or does matter make sense of sensation? Part 2. *Perception.* 18: 1–4.

Grillner, S., and Matsushima, T. (1991). The neural network underlying locomotion in lamprey synaptic and cellular mechanisms. Neuron 7: 1–15.

Gross, C. G., and Sergent, J. (1992). Face recognition. *Curr. Opin. Neurobiol.* 2: 156–161.

Hadders-Algra, M., Brogren, E., and Forssberg, H. (1997). Nature and nurture in the development of postural control in human infants. *Acta. Paediatr. Suppl.* 422: 48–53.

Hamburger, V., and Balaban, M. (1963). Observations and experiments on spontaneous rhythmical behavior in the chick embryo. *Dev. Biol.* 7: 533–545.

Hammer, M., and Menzel, R. (1995). Learning and memory in the honeybee. *J. Neurosci.* 15: 1617–1630.

Harris, D. F. (1894). The time-relations of the voluntary tetanns in man. *J. Physiol. (Lond.)* 17: 315–330.

Harris, J. E., and Whiting, H. P. W. (1954a). Structure and function in the locomotory system of the dogfish embryo. The myogenic stage of movement. *J. Physiol.* 501–524.

Harris, J. E., and Whiting, H. P. W. (1954b). Structure and functional feedback in the control of movement. *Trends Neurosc.* 7: 253–257.

Hartshorn, K., Rovee-Collier, C., Gerhardstein, P., Bhatt, R. S., Klein, P. J., Aaron, F., Wondoloski, T. L., and Wurtzel, N. (1998). Developmental changes in the specificity of memory over the first year of life. *Dev. Psychobiol.* 33: 61–78.

Hayhoe, M. M., Bensinger, D. G., and Ballard, D. H. (1998). Task constraints in visual working memory. *Vision Res.* 38: 125–137.

Hayman, L. A., Rexer, J. L., Pavol, M. A., Strite, D., and Meyers, C. A. (1998). Kluver-Bucy syndrome after bilateral selective damage of amygdala and its cortical connections. *J. Neuropsychiatry Clin. Neurosci.* 10: 354–358.

Heaton, J. T., Dooling, R. J., and Farabaugh, S. M. (1999). Effects of deafening on the calls and warble song of adult budgerigars (*Melopsittacus undulatus*). *J. Acoust. Soc. Am.* 105: 2010–2019.

Hebb, D. O. (1953). Heredity and environment in mammalian behavior. *Brit. J. Animal Behav.* 1: 43–47.

Heilman, K. M., and Gilmore, R. L. (1998). Cortical influences in emotion. *J. Clin. Neurophysiol.* 15: 409–423.

Hess, E. H. (1972). The natural history of imprinting. *Ann. NY Acad. Sci.* 193: 124–136.

Hess, R. W. (1957). *The Functional Organization of the Diencephalon.* New York: Grune and Stratton.

Hess R. W., and Rugger, M. (1943). Das subkortikale Zentrum der affektiven Abwehr-reaktion. *Helv. Physiol. Acta.* 1: 33–52.

Hikosaka, O. (1998). Neural systems for control of voluntary action—a hypothesis. *Adv. Biophys.* 35: 81–102.

Hildebrand, J. G. (1995). Analysis of chemical signals by nervous systems. *Proc. Natl. Acad. Sci. USA* 92: 67–74.

Hille, B. (1992). *Ionic Channels of Excitable Membranes,* 2d ed. New York: Sinauer Associates.

Hirose, H., and Gay, T. (1973). Laryngeal control in vocal attack. An electromyographic study. *Folia Phoniatr (Basel)* 25: 203–213.

Honda, K., and Kusakawa, N. (1997). Compatibility between auditory and articulatory representations of vowels. *Acta. Otolaryngol. Suppl. (Stockh.)* 532: 103–105.

Hubbard, T. L. (1996). The importance of a consideration of qualia to imagery and cognition. *Conscious Cogn.* 5: 327–358.

Hubel, D. H. (1988). *Eye, Brain, and Vision.* Scientific American Library Series, #22. New York: Freeman and Company.

Hubel, D. H., and Wiesel, T. N. (1963). Receptive fields of cells in striate cortex of very young, visually inexperienced kittens. *J. Neurophysiol.* 26: 994–1002.

Hubel, D. H., and Wiesel, T. N. (1974). Sequence regularity and geometry of orientation columns in the monkey striate cortex. *J. Comp. Neurol.* 158: 267–294.

Hubel, D. H., and Wiesel, T. N. (1977). Ferrier lecture: Functional architecture of macaque monkey visual cortex. *Proc. Roy. Soc. Serv. B.* 198: 1–59.

Hubel, D. H., and Wiesel, T. N. (1979). Brain mechanisms of vision. *Sci. Am.* 241: 150–162.

Hubel, D. H., Wiesel, T. N., and LeVay, S. (1976). Functional architecture of area 17 in normal and monocularly deprived macaque monkeys. *Cold Spring Harb. Symp. Quant. Biol.* 40: 581–589.

Hunsperger R. W. (1956). Role of substantia gricea centralis mesencephali in electrically induced rage reactions. *Folia Psychiat. (Amst.).* 19: 289–294.

Hutcheon, B., and Yarom, Y. (2000). Resonance, oscillation and intrinsic frequency preferences of neurons. *TINS* 23: 216–222.

Huxley A. (1980). *Reflections on muscle,* Princeton University Press, Princeton.

Ito, M. (1984). *The Cerebellum and Neural Control.* New York: Raven Press.

Iverson, P. and Kuhl, P. K. (1996). Influences of phonetic identification and category goodness on American listeners' perception of /r/ and /l/. *J. Acoust. Soc. Am.* 99: 1130–1140.

Iyengar, S., Viswanathan, S. S., and Bottjer, S. W. (1999). Development of topography within song control circuitry of zebra finches during the sensitive period for song learning. *J. Neurosci.* 19: 6037–6057.

James, W. (1950 [1890]). *Principles of Psychology.* New York: Dover.

Jankowska, E., and Edgley, S. (1993). Interactions between pathways controlling posture and gait at the level of spinal interneurons in the cat. *Prog. Brain Res.* 97: 161–171.

Jeannerod, M. (1986). Mechanisms of visuomotor coordination: A study in normal and brain-damaged subjects. *Neuropsychologia.* 24: 41–78.

Johnson, F., and Bottjer, S. W. (1993). Hormone-induced changes in identified cell populations of the higher vocal center in male canaries. *J. Neurobiol.* 24: 400–418.

Joliot, M., Ribary, U., and Llinás, R. (1994). Human oscillatory brain activity near 40 Hz coexists with cognitive temporal binding. *Proc. Natl. Acad. Sci. USA* 91: 11748–11751.

Jurgens, U. (1998). Neuronal control of mammalian vocalization, with special reference to the squirrel monkey. *Naturwissenschaften.* 85: 376–388.

Jurgens, U., and Zwirner, P. (1996). The role of the periaqueductal grey in limbic and neocortical vocal fold control. *Neuroreport.* 7: 2921–2923.

Jusczyk, P. W., and Bertoncini, J. (1988). Viewing the development of speech perception as an innately guided learning process. *Lang. Speech.* 31: 217–238.

Kahn, J. A., Roberts, A., and Kashin, S. M. (1982). The neuromuscular basis of swimming movements in embryos of the amphibian *Xenopus laevis. J. Exp. Biol.* 99: 175–184.

Kam, Y., Kim, D. Y., Koo, S. K., and Joe, C. O. (1998). Transfer of second messengers through gap junction connexin 43 channels reconstituted in liposomes. *Biochim. Biophys. Acta.* 1372: 384–388

Kandel, E. R., Schwartz, J. H., and Jessell, T. M. (eds.) (2000). *Principles of Neural Science,* 4th ed. New York: McGraw-Hill.

Kandler, K., and Katz, L. C. (1995). Neuronal coupling and uncoupling in the developing nervous system. *Curr. Opin. Neurobiol.* 5: 98–105.

Kant, I. (1781). *Critique of Pure Reason.* J. M. Meiklejohn (translator); Norman K. Smith, ed. St. Martin's Press, Inc. 1990

Kay, R. F., Cartmill, M., Balow, M. (1998). They hypoglossal canal and the origin of human vocal behavior. *Proc Natl Acad Sci USA.* 95: 5417–5419.

Kirk, D. L. (1998). *Volvox: Molecular-Genetic Origins of Multicellularity and Cellular Differentiation.* (Development and cell biology series). Cambridge: Cambridge University Press.

Kirzinger, A., and Jurgens, U. (1991). Vocalization-correlated single-unit activity in the brain stem of the squirrel monkey. *Exp. Brain Res.* 84: 545–560.

Kling, J. W., and Stevenson-Hinde, J. (1977). Development of song and reinforcing effects of song in female chaffinches. *Anim. Behav.* 25: 215–220.

Klüver, H., and Bucy, P. (1939). Preliminary analysis of functions of the temporal lobes in monkeys. *Arch. Neurol. Psychiat. (Chic.).* 42: 979–1000.

Konishi, M. (1989). Birdsong for neurobiologists. *Neuron* 3: 541–549.

Kretsinger R. H. (1997). EF-hands embrace. *Nat. Struct. Biol.* 4: 514–516.

Kretsinger, R. H. (1996). EF-hands reach out. *Nat. Struct. Biol.* 3: 12–15.

Krishtalka, L., Stucky, R. K., and Beard, K. C. (1990). The earliest fossil evidence for sexual dimorphism in primates. *Proc. Natl. Acad. Sci. USA.* 87: 5223–5226.

Kristofferson, A. B. (1984). Quantal and deterministic timing in human duration discrimination. *Ann. NY Acad. Sci.* 423: 3–15.

Kropotov, J. D., and Etlinger, S. C. (1999). Selection of actions in the basal ganglia-thalamocortical circuits: Review and model. *Int. J. Psychophysiol.* 31: 197–217.

Kuhl, P. K., Andruski, J. E., Christovich, I. A., Chistovich, L. A., Kozhevnikova, E. V., Ryskina, V. L., Stolyarova, E. I., Sundberg, U., Lacerda, F. (1997). Cross-language analysis of phonetic units in language addressed to infants. *Science.* 277: 684–686.

Kuhl, P. K. (2000) Language, mind, and brain: Experience alters perception. In M. S. Gazzaniga (ed.), *The New Cognitive Neurosciences,* 2nd edition, pp. 99–115. Cambridge, MA: MIT Press.

Kuroda, R., Yorimae, A., Yamada, Y., Furuta, Y., and Kim, A. (1995). Frontal cingulotomy reconsidered from a WGA-HRP and c-Fos study in cat. *Acta. Neurochir. Suppl. (Wien).* 64: 69–73.

Kutukca, Y., Marks, W. J. Jr, Goodin, D. S., and Aminoff, M. J. (1998). Cerebral accompaniments to simple and choice reaction tasks in Parkinson's disease. *Brain Res.* 799: 1–5.

LaBerge, S. and Rheingold, H. (1990). *Exploring the World of Lucid Dreaming.* New York: Ballantine.

Lamarre, Y., Montigny, C. de, Dumont, M., and Weiss, M. (1971). Harmaline-induced rhythmic activity of cerebellar and lower brain stem neurons. *Brain Res.* 32: 246–250.

Land, M. F. (1978). Animal eyes with mirror optics. *Sci. Am.* 239: 126–135.

Land, M. F. (1980). Compound eyes: Old and new optical mechanisms. *Nature.* 287: 681–686.

Land, M. F., and Fernald, R. D. (1992). The evolution of eyes. *Annu. Rev. Neurosc.* 15: 1–29.

Lang, E. J., Sugihara, I., and Llinás, R. (1996). GABAergic modulation of complex spike activity by the cerebellar nucleoolivary pathway in rat. *J. Neurophysiol.* 76: 255–275.

Lansner, A., Kotaleski, J. H., and Grillner, S. (1998). Modeling of the spinal neuronal circuitry underlying locomotion in a lower vertebrate. *Ann. NY Acad. Sci.* 860: 239–49.

Larson, C. R. (1985). The midbrain periaqueductal gray: A brainstem structure involved in vocalization. *J. Speech Hear. Res.* 28: 241–249.

Larson, C. R., Kistler, M. K. (1984). Periaqueductal gray neuronal activity associated with laryngeal EMG and vocalization of the awake monkey. *Neurosci Lett.* 46: 261–266.

Larson, C. R., and Kistler, M. K. (1986). The relationship of periaqueductal gray neurons to vocalization and laryngeal EMG in the behaving monkey. *Exp. Brain Res.* 63: 596–606.

Laurent, G. (1996). Dynamical representation of odors by oscillating and evolving neural assemblies. *Trends Neurosci.* 19: 489–496.

LeDoux, J. (1996) *The Emotional Brain.* New York: Simon and Schuster.

LeDoux, J. (1998). Fear and the brain: Where have we been, and where are we going? *Biol. Psychiatry.* 44: 1229–1238.

Leeds, S. (1993). Qualia, awareness, sellars. *Nous.* 27: 303–330.

Lehky S. R., and Sejnowski T. J. (1999). Seeing white: Qualia in the context of decoding population codes. *Neural Comput.* 11: 1261–1280.

Lengeler, J. W., Drews, G., and Schlegel, H. G. (eds.). (1999) *Biology of the Prokaryotes.* Boston: Blackwell Science Inc.

Llinás, R. (1974). La forme et la fonction des cellules nerveuses. *La Recherche.* 5: 232–240.

Llinás, R. (1981). Microphysiology of the cerebellum. In: *Handbook of Physiology,* vol. II, *The Nervous System,* part II, ed. V. B. Brooks. Bethesda, MD: American Physiology Society, pp. 831–976.

Llinás, R. (1987). "Mindness" as a functional state of the brain. In: *Mind Waves,* ed. C. Blakemore, S. A. Greenfield. Oxford: Basil Blackwell, pp. 339–358.

Llinás, R. (1988). The intrinsic electrophysiological properties of mammalian neurons: Insights into central nervous system function. *Science* 242: 1654–1664.

Llinás R. (1990). Intrinsic electrical properties of mammalian neurons and CNS function. In *Fidia Research Foundation Neuroscience Award Lectures,* Vol. 4. New York: Raven Press, pp. 175–194.

Llinás, R. (1991). The noncontinuous nature of movement execution. In: *Motor control: Concepts and Issues,* ed. D. R. Humphrey, H. J. Freund. New York: John Wiley & Sons, pp. 223–242.

Llinás, R., Grace, A. A., and Yarom, Y. (1991). In vitro neurons in mammalian cortical layer 4 exhibit intrinsic oscillatory activity in the 10-Hz to 50-Hz frequency range. *Proc. Natl. Acad. Sci. USA* 88: 897–901.

Llinás, R., and Pare, D. (1991). Of dreaming and wakefulness. *Neuroscience* 44: 521–535.

Llinás, R., and Ribary, U. (1993). Coherent 40-Hz oscillation characterizes dream state in humans. *Proc. Natl. Acad. Sci. USA* 90: 2078–2081.

Llinás, R., Ribary, U., and Tallal P. (1998). Dyschronic language-based learning disability. In *Basic Mechanisms in Cognition and Language,* ed. Von Euler et al. New York: Oxford.

Llinás, R., Ribary, U., Contreras, D., and Pedroarena, C. (1998). The neuronal basis for consciousness. *Phil. Trans. R. Soc. Lond. B* 353: 1841–1849.

Llinás, R. R., and Simpson, J. I. (1981). Cerebellar control of movement. In *Motor Coordination,* vol. 5. *Handbook of Behavioral Neurology,* ed. A. L. Towe and E. S. Luschel. New York: Plenum Press, pp. 231–302.

Llinás R., and Volkind, R. A. (1973). The olivo-cerebellar system: Functional properties as revealed by harmaline-induced tremor. *Exp. Brain Res.* 18: 69–87.

Llinás R., Walton, K., Hillman, D. E., and Sotelo, C. (1975). Inferior olive: Its role in motor learning. *Science* 190: 1230–1231.

Llinás, R. and Welsh, J. P. (1993). On the cerebellum and motor learning. *Curr. Opinion Neurobiol.* 3: 958–965.

Llinás R., and Yarom, Y. (1981a). Electrophysiology of mammalian inferior olivary neurons in vitro. Different types of voltage-dependent ionic conductances. *J. Physiol. (Lond.).* 315: 549–567.

Llinás R., and Yarom, Y. (1981b). Properties and distribution of ionic conductances generating electroresponsiveness of inferior olivary neurons in vitro. *J. Physiol. (Lond.)* 315: 569–584.

Locke, J. L. (1990). Structure and stimulation in the ontogeny of spoken language. *Dev. Psychobiol.* 23: 621–643.

Logan, J. S., Lively, S. E., and Pisoni, D. B. (1991). Training Japanese listeners to identify English /r/ and /l/: A first report. *J. Acoust. Soc. Am.* 89: 874–886.

Loi, P., Saunders, R., Young, D., and Tublitz, N. (1996). Peptidergic regulation of chromatophore function in the European cuttlefish *Sepia officinalis*. *J. Exp. Biol.* 199: 1177–1187.

Lorenz, K. (1935). Der kumpan in der umwelt des vogels. *J. Ornithol.* 83: 137–213.

Lorenz, K. (1937). Uber die bildung des instinktbegriffes. *Naturwiss Enschaften.* 25: 289–300.

Lutzenberger, W., Pulvermuller, F., Elbert, T., and Birbaumer, N. (1995). Visual stimulation alters local 40-Hz responses in humans: An EEG study. *Neurosci. Lett.* 183: 39–42.

MacDougall-Shackleton, S. A., Hulse, S. H., and Ball, G. F. (1998). Neural correlates of singing behavior in male zebra finches (*Taeniopygia guttata*). *J. Neurobiol.* 36: 421–430.

MacNeilage, P. F. (1994). Prolegomena to a theory of the sound pattern of the first spoken language. *Phonetica* 51: 184–194.

MacNeilage, P. F. (1998). The frame/content theory of evolution of speech production. *Behav. Brain Sci.* 21: 499–511.

Makarenko, V., and Llinás, R. (1998). Experimentally determined chaotic phase synchronization in a neuronal system. *Proc. Natl. Acad. Sci. USA* 95: 15747–15752.

Marder, E. (1998). From biophysics to models of network function. *Annu. Rev. Neurosci.* 21: 25–45.

Marder, E., Abbott, L. F., Turrigiano, G. G., Liu, Z., and Golowasch, J. (1996). Memory from the dynamics of intrinsic membrane currents. *Proc. Natl. Acad. Sci. USA.* 93: 13481–13486.

Margulis, L., and Olendzenski, L. (eds.). (1992). *Environmental Evolution: Effects of the Origin and Evolution of Life on Planet Earth.* Cambridge: MIT Press.

Margulis, L., and Sagan, D. (1985). Order amidst animalcules: The Protoctista kingdom and its undulipodiated cells. *Biosystems.* 18: 141–147.

Marsden, C. D., Rothwell, J. C., and Day, B. L. (1984). The use of peripheral feedback in the control of movement. *Trends Neurosci.* 7: 253–257.

Marshall, J., and Geoffrey-Walsh, E. (1956). Physiological tremor. *J. Neurol. Neurosurg. Psychiat.* 19: 260–267.

Mazza, E., Nunez-Abades, P. A., Spielmann, J. M., and Cameron, W. E. (1992). Anatomical and electrotonic coupling in developing genioglossal motoneurons of the rat. *Brain Res.* 598: 127–137.

McCulloch, W. S. (1965). *Embodiments of Mind.* Cambridge, MA: MIT Press.

McPeek, R. M., Maljkovic, V., and Nakayama, K. (1999). Saccades require focal attention and are facilitated by a short-term memory system. *Vision Res.* 39: 1555–1566.

Menzel, R., and Muller, U. (1996). Learning and memory in honeybees: From behavior to neural substrates. *Annu. Rev. Neurosci.* 19: 379–404.

Miklos, G. L. (1993). Molecules and cognition: The latterday lessons of levels, language, and lac. Evolutionary overview of brain structure and function in some vertebrates and invertebrates. *J. Neurobiol.* 24: 842–890.

Miles, F. A. (1999). Short-latency visual stabilization mechanisms that help to compensate for translational disturbances of gaze. *Ann. NY Acad. Sci.* 871: 260–271.

Millar, R. H. (1971). The biology of ascidians. *Adv. Mar. Biol.* 9: 1–100.

Miller, R. J. (1992). Ingested ethanol as a factor in double vision. *Ann. NY Acad. Sci.* 654: 489–491.

Millican, P., and Clark A., (eds). (1996). *Machines and Thought: The Legacy of Alan Turing* (Mind Association Occasional Series), vol. 1. Oxford: Clarendon Press.

Milner, B. (1962). Les troubles de la mémoire accompagnant les lésions hippocampiques bilatérales. In: *Physiologie de l'Hippocampe, Colloques Internationaux* No. 107 (Paris, C.N.R.S.), pp. 257–272. [English translation (1965). In: *Cognitive Processes and the Brain,* ed. P. M. Milner and S. Glickman, pp. 97–111. Princeton, NJ: Van Nostrand]

Milner, B., Squire, B. R., and Kandel, E. R. (1998). Cognitive neuroscience and the study of memory. *Neuron* 20: 445–468.

Mitcheson, J. S., Hancox, J. C., and Levi, A. J. (1998). Cultured adult cardiac myocytes: Future applications, culture methods, morphological and electrophysiological properties. *Cardiovasc. Res.* 39: 280–300.

Molotchnikoff, S., and Shumikhina, S. (1996). The lateral posterior-pulvinar complex modulation of stimulus-dependent oscillations in the cat visual cortex. *Vision Res.* 36: 2037–2046.

Montague, P. R., Dayan, P., Person, C., and Sejnowski, T. J. (1995). Bee foraging in uncertain environments using predictive hebbian learning. *Nature.* 377: 725–728.

de Montigny, C., and Lamarre, Y. (1973). Rhythmic activity induced by harmaline in the olivo-cerebellar-bulbar system of the cat. *Brain Res.* 53: 81–95.

Mooney, R. (1999). Sensitive periods and circuits for learned birdsong. *Curr. Opin. Neurobiol.* 9: 121–127.

Moray, N. (1972). Visual mechanisms in the copepod *Copilia. Perception.* 1: 193–207.

Morrow, N. S., Grijalva C. V., Geiselman, P. J., and Novin, D. (1993). Effects of amygdaloid lesions on gastric erosion formation during exposure to activity-stress. *Physiol. Behav.* 53: 1043–1048.

Mortin, L. I., and Stein, P. S. (1989). Spinal cord segments containing key elements of the central pattern generators for three forms of scratch reflex in the turtle. *Neuroscience* 9: 2285–2296.

Mountcastle, V. B. (1979). An organizing principle for cerebral function: The unit module and the distributed system. In: *The Neurosciences. Fourth Study Program.* Cambridge: MIT Press, pp. 21–42.

Mountcastle, V. B. (1997). The columnar organization of the neocortex. *Brain* 120: 701–722.

Mountcastle, V. B. (1998). *Perceptual Neuroscience. The Cerebral Cortex.* Cambridge: Harvard University Press.

Nespor, A. A., Lukazewicz, M. J., Dooling, R. J., and Ball, G. F. (1996). Testosterone induction of male-like vocalizations in female budgerigars (*Melopsittacus undulatus*). *Horm. Behav.* 30: 162–169.

Neuenschwander, S., and Singer, W. (1996). Long-range synchronization of oscillatory light responses in the cat retina and lateral geniculate nucleus. *Nature* 379: 728–732.

Nichols, T. R. (1994). A biomechanical perspective on spinal mechanisms of coordinated muscular action: An architecture principle. *Acta. Anat. (Basel).* 151: 1–13.

Nordeen, E. J., Grace, A., Burek, M. J., and Nordeen, K. W. (1992). Sex-dependent loss of projection neurons involved in avian song learning. *J. Neurobiol.* 23: 671–679.

Nordeen, K. W., and Nordeen, E. J. (1992). Auditory feedback is necessary for the maintenance of stereotyped song in adult zebra finches. *Behav. Neural Biol.* 57: 58–66.

Nordeen, K. W., and Nordeen, E. J. (1993). Long-term maintenance of song in adult zebra finches is not affected by lesions of a forebrain region involved in song learning. *Behav. Neural. Biol.* 59: 79–82.

Nordeen, K. W., and Nordeen, E. J. (1997). Anatomical and synaptic substrates for avian song learning. *J. Neurobiol.* 33: 532–548.

Nottebohm, F. (1980). Testosterone triggers growth of brain vocal control nuclei in adult female canaries. *Brain Res.* 189: 429–436.

Nottebohm, F. (1981a). Gonadal hormones induce dendritic growth in the adult avian brain. *Science* 214: 202–204.

Nottebohm, F. (1981b). A brain for all seasons: Cyclical anatomical changes in song control nuclei of the canary brain. *Science* 214: 1368–1370.

Nottebohm, F., and Arnold, A. P. (1976). Sexual dimorphism in vocal control areas of the songbird brain. *Science* 194: 211–213.

Nottebohm, F., Nottebohm, M. E., and Crane, L. (1986). Developmental and seasonal changes in canary song and their relation to changes in the anatomy of song-control nuclei. *Behav. Neural. Biol.* 46: 445–471.

Nowak, M. A., and Krakauer, D. C. (1999). The evolution of language. *Proc. Natl. Acad. Sci. USA* 96: 8028–8033.

Nunez, A., Amzica, F., and Steriade, M. (1992). Voltage-dependent fast (20–40 Hz) oscillations in long-axoned neocortical neurons. *Neuroscience* 51: 7–10.

O'Donovan, M. J. (1987). Developmental approaches to the analysis of vertebrate central pattern generators. *J. Neurosci. Methods* 21: 275–286.

Olanow, C. W., and Tatton, W. G. (1999). Etiology and pathogenesis of Parkinson's disease. *Annu. Rev. Neurosci.* 22: 123–144.

Ono, T., Fukuda, M., Nishino, H., Sasaki, K., and Muramoto, K. I. (1983). Amygdaloid neuronal responses to complex visual stimuli in an operant feeding situation in the monkey. *Brain Res. Bull.* 11: 515–518.

Ostry, D. J., Feldman, A. G., and Flanagan, J. R. (1991). Kinematics and control of frog hindlimb movements. *J. Neurophysiol.* 65: 547–562.

Pankesepp, J. (1998). *Affective Neuroscience.* Oxford: Oxford University Press.

Pantev, C., Makeig, S., Hoke, M., Galambos, R., Hampson, S., and Gallen, C. (1991). Human auditory evoked gamma-band magnetic fields. *Proc. Natl. Acad. Sci. USA* 88: 8996–9000.

Parker, G. H. (1919). *The Elementary Nervous System.* Philadelphia: Lippincott.

Passingham, R. E. (1981). Broca's area and the origins of human vocal skill. *Philos. Trans. R. Soc. Lond. B. Biol. Sci.* 292: 167–175.

Paulesu, E., Frith, C. D., and Frackowiak, R. S. (1993). The neural correlates of the verbal component of working memory. *Nature.* 362: 342–345.

Pedroarena, C. M., and Llinás, R. (1998). Dendritic calcium conductance generate high frequency oscillations in thalamocortical neurons. *Proc. Natl. Acad. Sci. USA* 94: 724–728.

Pellionisz, A., and Llinás, R. (1979). Brain modeling by tensor network theory and computer simulation. The cerebellum: Distributed processor for predictive coordination. *Neuroscience* 4: 323–348.

Pellionisz, A., and Llinás, R. (1980). Tensorial approach to the geometry of brain function: Cerebellar coordination via metric tensor. *Neuroscience* 5: 1125–1136.

Pellionisz, A., and Llinás, R. (1982). Space-time representation in the brain. The cerebellum as a predictive space-time metric tensor. *Neuroscience* 7: 2949–2970.

Pellionisz, A., and Llinás, R. (1985). Tensor network theory of the metaorganization of functional geometries in the CNS. *Neuroscience* 16: 245–273.

Penfield, W., and Milner, B. (1958). Memory deficits induced by bilateral lesions in the hippocampal zone. *Am. Med. Assoc. Arch. Neurol. Psychiatry* 79: 475–497.

Penfield, W., and Rasmussen, T. (1950). *The Cerebral Cortex of Man.* New York: MacMillan.

Penn, A. A., Riquelme, P. A., Feller, M. B., and Shatz, C. J. (1998). Competition in retinogeniculate patterning driven by spontaneous activity. *Science* 279: 2108–2112.

Perrett D. I., Rolls, E. T., and Caan, W. (1982). Visual neurons responsive to faces in the monkey temporal cortex. *Exp. Brain Res.* 47: 329–342.

Persinger, M. A., and Makarec, K. (1992). The feeling of a presence and verbal meaningfulness in context of temporal lobe function: Factor analytic verification of the muses? *Brain Cogn.* 20: 217–226.

Pietrobon, D., Di Virgilio, F., and Pozzan, T. (1990). Structural and functional aspects of calcium homeostasis in eukaryotic cells. *Eur. J. Biochem.* 193: 599–622.

Pitts, J. D., and Simms, J. W. (1977). Permeability of junctions between animal cells: Intercellular transfer of nucleotides but not of macromolecules. *Ex. Cell Res.* 104: 153–163.

Plavcan, J. M. (1993). Canine size and shape in male anthropoid primates. *Am. J. Phys. Anthropol.* 92: 201–216.

Plum, F., Schiff, N., Ribary, U., and Llinás, R. (1998). Coordinated expression in chronically unconscious persons. *Philos. Trans. R. Soc. Lond. B Biol. Sci.* 353: 1929–1933.

Posner, M. I., and Raichle, M. (1995). *Images of Mind.* New York: W. H. Freeman.

Rainville, P., Duncan, G. H., Price, D. D., Carrier, B., and Bushnell, M. C. (1997). Pain affect encoded in human anterior cingulate but not somatosensory cortex. *Science* 277: 968–971.

Ramachandran, V. S., Clarke, P. G., and Whitteridge, D. (1977). Cells selective to binocular disparity in the cortex of newborn lambs. *Nature* 268: 333–335.

Ramachandran, V. S., Tyler, C. W., Gregory, R. L., Rogers-Ramachandran, D., Duensing S., Pillsbury, C., and Ramachandran, C. (1996). Rapid adaptive camouflage in tropical flounders. *Nature* 379: 815–818.

Ramón y Cajal (1911). *Histologie du systeme nervex de l'homme et des vertebres.* Paris: Maloine.

Rasika, S., Alvarez-Buylla, A., and Nottebohm, F. (1999). BDNF mediates the effects of testosterone on the survival of new neuronsin an adult brain. *Neuron* 22: 53–62.

Rasika, S., Nottebohm, F., and Alvarez, Buylla, A. (1994). Testosterone increases the recruitment and/or survival of new high vocal center neurons in adult female canaries. *Proc. Natl. Acad. Sci. USA.* 91: 7854–7858.

Ray, A., Henke, P. G., Gulati, K., and Sen, P. (1993). The amygdaloid complex, corticotropin releasing factor and stress-induced gastric ulcerogenesis in rats. *Brain Res.* 624: 286–290.

Redgrave, P., Prescott, T. J., and Gurney, K. (1999). The basal ganglia: A vertebrate solution to the selection problem? *Neuroscience* 89: 1009–1023.

Reed, J. M., Squire, L. R., Patalano, A. L., Smith, E. E., and Jonides, J. (1999). Learning about categories that are defined by impaired declarative memory. *Behav. Neurosci.* 113: 411–419.

Ribary, U., Ioannides, A. A., Singh, K. D., Hasson, R., Bolton J. P. R., Lado, R., Mogilner, A., and Llinás, R. (1991). Magnetic field tomography (MFT) of coherent thalamo-cortical 40-Hz oscillations in humans. *Proc. Natl. Acad. Sci. USA.* 88: 11037–11041.

Ridley, M. (1996). *Evolution,* 2d ed. Boston: Blackwell Science.

Ringham, G. L. (1975). Localization and electrical characteristics of a giant synapse in the spinal cord of the lamprey. *J. Physiol. (Lond.)* 251: 395–407.

Robertson, M. M., and Stern, J. S. (1997). Gilles de la Tourette syndrome. *Br. J. Hosp. Med.* 58: 253–256.

Roelofs, W. L. (1995). Chemistry of sex attraction. *Proc. Natl. Acad. Sci. USA.* 92: 44–49.

Rolls, E. T. (1992). Neurophysiological mechanisms underlying face processing within and beyond the temporal cortical visual areas. *Phil. Trans. R. Soc. Lond. B Biol. Sci.* 335: 11–20.

Rolls E. T. (1999). *The Brain and Emotion.* Oxford: Oxford University Press.

Romer, A. S. (1969). Vertebrate history with special reference to factors related to cerebellar evolution. In *Neurobiology of Cerebellar Evolution and Development,* ed. R. Llinás. Chicago: Amer. Med. Assn., pp. 1–18.

Rosenzweig, M. R., Leiman, A. L., and Breedlove, S. M. (1999). *Biological Psychology: An Introduction to Behavioral, Cognitive and Clinical Neuroscience.* Sunderland, Mass.: Sinauer.

Routtenberg, A. (1978). *The Reward System of the Brain.* Readings from *Scientific American* Magazine. New York: W.H. Freeman.

Rovee-Collier, C. (1997). Dissociations in infant memory: Rethinking the development of implicit and explicit memory. *Psychol. Rev.* 104: 467–498.

Saba, P. R., Dastur, K., Keshavan, M. S., and Katerji, M. A. (1998). Obsessive-compulsive disorder, Tourette's syndrome, and basal ganglia pathology on MRI. *J. Neuropsychiatry Clin. Neurosci.* 10: 116–117.

Sacks, O. (1996). The last hippie. In: *An Anthropologist on Mars: Seven Paradoxical Tales.* New York: Vintage Books.

Saint-Cyr, J. A., Taylor, A. E., and Nicholson, K. (1995). Behavior and the basal ganglia. *Adv. Neurol.* 65: 1–28.

Saper, C. B. (1996). Role of the cerebral cortex and striatum in emotional motor response. *Prog. Brain Res.* 107: 537–550.

Savander, V., Go, C. G., Ledoux, J. E., and Pitkanen, A. (1996). Intrinsic connections of the rat amygdaloid complex: Projections originating in the accessory basal nucleus. *J. Comp. Neurol.* 374: 291–313.

Schacter, D. L. (1987). Implicit memory: History and current status. *J Exp. Psychol. Learning, Memory, and Cogn.* 13: 501–518.

Schacter, D. L., and Buckner, R. L. (1998). On the relations among priming, conscious recollection, and intentional retrieval: Evidence from neuroimaging research. *Neurobiol. Learn. Mem.* 70: 284–303.

Schacter D. L., Buckner, R. L., and Koutstaal, W. (1998). Memory, consciousness and neuroimaging. *Philos. Trans. R. Soc. Lond. B Biol. Sci.* 353: 1861–1878.

Schäfer, E. A. (1886). On the rhythm of muscular response to volitional impulses in man. *J. Physiol. (Lond.)* 7: 111–117.

Scharff, C., and Nottebohm, F. (1991). A comparative study of the behavioral deficits following lesions of various parts of the zebra finch song system: Implications for vocal learning. *J. Neurosci.* 11: 2896–2913.

Schiff, N., Ribary, U., Plum, F., and Llinás, R. (1999). Words without mind. *J. Cogn. Neurosci.* 11: 650–656.

Schlinger B. A., and Arnold, A. P. (1991). Androgen effects on the development of the zebra finch song system. *Brain Res.* 561: 99–105.

Schotland, J. L., and Rymer, W. Z. (1993). Wipe and flexion reflexes of the frog. II. Response to perturbations. *J. Neurophysiol.* 69: 1736–1748.

Schwartz-Giblin, S., and Pfaff, D. W. (1985–86). Hypothalamic output controlling reticulospinal and vestibulospinal systems important for emotional behavior. *Int. J. Neurol.* 19–20: 89–110.

Scoville, W. B. (1954). The limbic lobe in man. *J. Neurosurg.* 11: 64–66.

Scoville, W. B., and Milner, B. (1957). Loss of recent memory after bilateral hippocampal lesions. *J. Neurol. Neurosurg. Psychiatry* 20: 11–21.

Searle, J. R. (1992). *The Rediscovery of Mind.* Cambridge: MIT Press.

Searle, J. R. (1998). How to study consciousness scientifically. *Philos. Trans. R. Soc. Lond. B Biol. Sci.* 353: 1935–1942.

Shapovalov, A. I. (1977). Interneuronal synapses with electrical and chemical mechanisms of transmission and the evolution of the central nervous system. *Zh. Evol. Biokhim. Fiziol.* 13: 621–632. [Article in Russian]

Shashar, N., Rutledge, P., and Cronin, T. (1996). Polarization vision in cuttlefish in a concealed communication channel? *J. Exp. Biol.* 199: 2077–2084.

Sherk, H. and Stryker, M. P. (1976). Quantitative study of cortical orientation selectivity in visually inexperienced kitten. *J. Neurophysiol.* 39: 63–70.

Sherrington, C. S. (1910). In: *Tendon Phenomenon and Spasm in System of Medicine,* ed. T. C. Allbut and H. D. Rolleston, pp. 290–304. London: MacMillan.

Sherrington, C. S. (1941). Man on his nature. In: *Gifford Lectures at Edinburgh in 1937,* chapter 12. The MacMillan Co., Cambridge, England, University Press.

Sherrington, C. S. (1948). *The Integrative Action of the Nervous System.* New York: Yale University Press.

Shipley, M. T., Murphy, A. Z., Rizvi, T. A., Ennis, M., and Behbehani, M. M. (1996). Olfaction and brainstem circuits of reproductive behavior in the rat. *Prog. Brain Res.* 107: 355–377.

Shors, T. J., and Matzel, L. D. (1997). Long-term potentiation: What's learning got to do with it? *Behav. Brain Sci.* 20: 597–614; discussion, 614–655.

Sierra, M., and Berrios, G. E. (1998). Depersonalization: Neurobiological perspectives. *Biol. Psychiatry* 44: 898–908.

Simpson, I., Rose, B., and Loewenstein, W. R. (1977). Size limit of molecules permeating the junctional membrane channels. *Science* 195: 294–296.

Singer, W. (1995). Development and plasticity of cortical processing architectures. *Science* 270: 758–764.

Skinner B. F. (1986) The evolution of verbal behavior. *J. Exp. An. Behav.* 45: 115–122.

Smart J. J. C. (1959) Sensations and brain processes. *Philos. Rev.* 68: 141–156.

Smith, G. T., Brenowitz, E. A., and Wingfield, J. C. (1997). Roles of photoperiod and testosterone in seasonal plasticity of the avian song control system. *J. Neurobiol.* 32: 426–442.

Smith, O. A., and deVito, J. L. (1984). Central neural integration for the control of autonomic responses associated with emotion. *Annu. Rev. Neurosci.* 7: 43–65.

Smith, S. S. (1998). Step cycle-related oscillatory properties of inferior olivary neurons recorded in ensembles. *Neuroscience* 82: 69–81.

Smith, Y., Bevan, M. D., Shink, E., and Bolam, J. P. (1998). Microcircuitry of the direct and indirect pathways of the basal ganglia. *Neuroscience* 86: 353–387.

Sokolov, A., Lutzenberger, W., Pavlova, M., Preissl, H., Braun, C., and Birbaumer, N. (1999). Gamma-band MEG activity to coherent motion depends on task-driven attention. *NeuroReport* 10: 1997–2000.

Sommerhoff, G., and MacDorman, K. (1994). An account of consciousness in physical and functional terms: A target for research in the neurosciences. *Integr. Physiol. Behav. Sci.* 29: 151–181.

Spyer, K. M. (1989). Neural mechanisms involved in cardiovascular control during affective behaviour. *Trends Neurosci.* 12: 506–513.

Stanford, L. R. (1987). Conduction velocity variations minimize conduction time differences among retinal ganglion cell axons. *Science* 238: 358–360.

Stein, P. S. (1983). The vertebrate scratch reflex. *Symp. Soc. Exp. Biol.* 37: 383–403.

Stein, P. S. (1989). Spinal cord circuits for motor pattern selection in the turtle. *Ann. NY Acad. Sci.* 563: 1–10.

Stein, P. S. G. (1984). Central pattern generators in the spinal cord. In: *Handbook of the Spinal Cord*, vols. 2 and 3: *Anatomy and Physiology*, ed. R A Davidoff. New York: Marcel Dekker, pp. 647–672

Stein P. S. G., Mortin L. I., and Robertson G. A. (1986). The forms of a task and their blends. In: *Neurobiology of Vertebrate Locomotion*, ed. S. Grillner, P. S. G. Stein, D. G. Stuart, H. Forssberg, R. M. Herman. London: Macmillan Press.

Steriade, M. (1991). Alertness, quiet sleep, dreaming. In: *Cerebral Cortex,* ed. A. Peters and E. G. Jones. eds. Vol. 9, *Normal and Altered States of Function,* New York: Plenum, pp. 279–357.

Steriade, M., Dossi, R. C., Pare, D., and Oakson, G. (1991). Fast oscillations (20–40 Hz) in thalamocortical systems and their potentiation by meopontine cholinergic nuclei in the cat. *Proc. Natl. Acad. Sci. USA.* 88: 4396–4400.

Steriade, M., and Amzica, F. (1996). Intracortical and corticothalamic coherency of fast spontaneous oscillations. Proc. Natl. Acad. Sci. USA. 93: 2533–2538.

Steriade, M., Contreras, D., Amzica, F., and Timofeev, I. (1996). Synchronization of fast (30–40 Hz) spontaneous oscillations in intrathalamic and thalamocortical networks. *J. Neurosci.* 16: 2788–2808.

Stock, D. W., Weiss, K. M., and Zhao, Z. (1997). Patterning of the mammalian dentition in development and evolution. *Bioessays* 19: 481–490.

Stoner, D. S. (1994). Larvae of a colonial ascidian use a non-contact mode of substratum selection on a coral reef. *Mar. Biol.* 121: 319–326.

Stryer, L. (1987). The molecules of visual excitation. *Scientific American* 257: 42–50.

Sudakov, K. V. (1997). Effects of acute emotional stress on the brain and autonomic variables. *Baillieres Clin. Neurol.* 6: 261–274.

Sugihara, I., Lang, E. J., and Llinás, R. (1993). Uniform olivocerebellar conduction time underlies Purkinje cell complex spike synchronicity in the rat cerebellum. *J. Physiol. (Lond.)* 470: 243–271.

Sussman, J. E., and Lauckner-Moreno, V. J. (1995). Further tests of the "perceptual magnet effect" in the perception of (i). *J. Acoust. Soc. Amer.* V. 34 Abs, 129th Annual Meeting.

Suthers, R. A. (1997). Peripheral control and lateralization of birdsong. *J. Neurobiol.* 33: 632–652.

Suthers, R. A., Goller, F., and Pytte, C. (1999). The neuromuscular control of birdsong. *Philos. Trans. R. Soc. Lond. B Biol. Sci.* 354: 927–939.

Svane, I. B., and Young, C. M. (1989). The ecology and behaviour of ascidian larvae. *Ocean Mar. Biol. Annu. Rev.* 27: 45–90.

Tchernichovski, O., and Nottebohm, F. (1998). Social inhibition of song imitation among sibling male zebra finches. *Proc. Natl. Acad. Sci. USA* 95: 8951–8956.

Tinbergen, N. (1951). *The Study of Instinct.* Oxford: Oxford University Press.

Tinbergen, N. (1966). *Animal Behavior.* New York: Time Life.

Tolle, T. R., Kaufmann, T., Siessmeier, T., Lautenbacher, S., Berthele, A., Munz, F., Zieglgansberger, W., Willoch, F., Schwaiger, M., Conrad, B., and Bartenstein, P. (1999). Region-specific encoding of sensory and affective components of pain in the human brain: A positron emission tomography correlation analysis. *Ann. Neurol.* 45: 40–47.

Tonomi, G., Sporns, O., and Edelman, G. M. (1992). Reentry and the problem of integrating multiple cortical areas: Simulation of dynamic intgration in the visual system. *Cerebral Cortex* 2: 310–335.

Tovee, M. J., Rolls, E. T., and Azzopardi, P. (1994). Translation invariance in the responses to faces of single neurons in the temporal visual cortical areas of the alert macaque. *J. Neurophysiol.* 72: 1049–1060.

Travis, C. E. (1929). Excitation as the physiological basis for tremor: A biophysical study of the oscillatory properties of mammalian central neurones in vitro. In: *Movement Disorders: Tremor,* ed. L. J. Findley and R. Capildeo. London: MacMillan, pp. 165–182.

Treede, R. D., Kenshalo, D. R., Gracely, R. H., and Jones, A. K. (1999). The cortical representation of pain. *Pain* 79: 105–111.

Trimble, M. R., Mendez, M. F., and Cummings, J. L. (1997). Neuropsychiatric symptoms from the temporolimbic lobes. *J. Neuropsychiatry Clin. Neurosci.* 9: 429–438.

Tulving, E. (1983). *Elements of Episodic Memory.* Oxford: Clarendon Press.

Tulving, E., and Schacter, D. L. (1990). Priming and human memory systems. *Science* 247: 301–306.

Turing, A. M. (1947). Lecture to the London mathematical society on 20 February 1947. *MD Comput.* 12: 390–397.

Ujhelyi, M. (1996). Is there any intermediate stage between animal communication and language? *J. Theor. Biol.* 180: 71–76.

Vallbo Å. B., and Wessberg, J. (1993). Organization of motor output in slow finger movements in man. *J. Physiol. (Lond.),* 469: 673–691.

Velasco, J. M., and Fernandez de Molina, A. (1988). Unitary activity in the suprarhinal cortex of the rat and its modulation after lateral amygdala stimulation. *Exp. Neurol.* 99: 447–453.

Velasco, J. M., Fernandez de Molina, A., and Perez, D. (1989). Suprarhinal cortex response to electrical stimulation of the lateral amygdala nucleus in the rat. *Exp. Brain Res.* 74: 168–172.

Verfaellie, M., and Keane, M. M. (1997). The neural basis of aware and unaware forms of memory. *Semin. Neurol.* 17: 153–161.

Verhaegen, M. (1995). Aquatic ape theory, speech origins, and brain differences with apes and monkeys. *Med. Hypotheses* 44: 409–413.

Vicario, D. S. (1994). Motor mechanisms relevant to auditory-vocal interactions in songbirds. *Brain Behav. Evol.* 44: 265–278.

Villablanca, J., and Riobo, F. (1970). Electroencephalographic and behavioral effects of harmaline in intact cats and in cats with chronic mesencephalic transection. *Psychopharmacologia* 17: 302–313.

Villee, C. A., and Dethier, V. G. (1971). *Biological Principles and Processes.* Philadelphia: W.B. Saunders.

Volkmann, J., Joliot, M., Mogilner, A., Ioannides A. A., Lado, F., Fazzini, E., Ribary, U., and Llinás, R. (1996). Central motor loop oscillations in parkinsonian resting tremor revealed by magnetoencephalography. *Neurology* 46: 1359–1370.

Von Frisch, K. (1994). [The "language" of bees and its utilization in agriculture. 1946] *Experientia* 50: 406–413.

Waddington, K. D., Nelson, C. M., and Page, R. E. (1998). Effects of pollen quality and genotype on the dance of foraging honey bees. *Anim. Behav.* 56: 35–39.

Wagner, A. D., Gabrieli, J. D. (1998) On the relationship between recognition familiarity and perceptual fluency: evidence for distinct mnemonic processes. *Acta Psychol (Amst).* 98: 211–230.

Ward, J. M. (1994). The auditory-vocal-respiratory axis in birds. *Brain Behav. Evol.* 44: 192–209.

Walton, K. D., and Navarrete, R. (1991). Postnatal changes in motoneurone electrotonic coupling studied in the in vitro rat lumbar spinal cord. *J. Physiol. (Lond.)* 433: 283–305.

Weinstock, V. M., Weinstock, D. J., and Kraft, S. P. (1998). Screening for childhood strabismus by primary care physicians. *Can. Fam. Physician* 44: 337–343.

Weiskrantz, L. (1956). Behavioral changes associated with ablation of the amygdaloidcomplex in monkeys. *J. Comp. Physiol. Psychol.* 49: 381–391.

Weiskrantz, L. (1990). Some contributions of neuropsychology of vision and memory to the problem of consciousness. In: *Consciousness and Contemporary Science,* ed. A. Marcel and E. Bisiach. (New York: Oxford University Press), pp. 183–197.

Welsh, J. P. (1998). Systemic harmaline blocks associative and motor learning by the actions of the inferior olive. *Eur. J. Neurosci.* 10: 3307–3320.

Welsh, J. P., Lang, E. J., Sugihara, I., and Llinás, R. (1995). Dynamic organization of motor control within the olivocerebellar system. *Nature* 374: 453–457.

Welsh, J. P., and Llinás, R. (1997). Some organizing principles for the control of movement based on olivocerebellar physiology. *Prog. Brain Res.* 114: 449–461.

Wenk, G. L. (1997). The nucleus basalis magnocellularis cholinergic system: One hundred years of progress. *Neurobiol. Learn. Mem.* 67: 85–95.

Werker, J. F., and Tees, R. C. (1999). Influences on infant speech processing: Toward a new synthesis. *Annu. Rev. Psychol.* 50: 509–535.

Wessberg, J., and Vallbo, Å. B. (1995). Human muscle spindle afferent activity in relation to visual and control in precision finger movements. *J. Physiol. (Lond.)* 482: 225–233.

Wexler, K. (1990). Innateness and maturation in linguistic development. *Dev. Psychobiol.* 23: 645–660.

Whaling, C. S., Solis, M. M., Doupe, A. J., Soha, J. A., and Marler, P. (1997). Acoustic and neural bases for innate recognition of song. *Proc. Natl. Acad. Sci. USA.* 94: 12694–12698.

Whelan, P. J. (1996). Control of locomotion in the decerebrate cat. *Prog. Neurobiol.* 49: 481–515.

Whiten, A., Goodall, J., McGrew, W. C., Nishida, T., Reynolds, V., Sugiyama, Y., Tutin, C. E. G., Wrangham, R. W., and Boesch, C. (1999). Cultures in chimpanzees. *Nature* 399: 682–685.

Whittington, M. A., Traub, R. D., and Jefferys, J. G. (1995). Synchronized oscillations in interneuron networks driven by metabotropic glutamate receptor activation. Nature. 373: 612–615.

Wiesel T. N., and Hubel, D. H. (1974). Ordered arrangement of orientation columns in monkeys lacking visual experience. *J. Comp. Neurol.* 158: 307–318.

Wiklund Fernstrom, K., Wessberg, J., Olausson, H., and Vallbo, A. (1999). Our second touch system: Receptive field properties of unmyelinated tactile afferents in man. *Acta Physiol. Scand.* 167: A26.

Wild, J. M. (1997a). Neural pathways for the control of birdsong production. *J. Neurobiol.* 33: 653–670.

Wild, J. M. (1997b). Functional anatomy of neural pathways contributing to the control of song production in birds. *Eur. J. Morphol.* 35: 303–325.

Williams, R. J. (1998). Calcium: Outside/inside homeostasis and signaling. *Biochim. Biophys. Acta.* 1448: 153–165.

Willis, M. A., and Arbas, E. A. (1991). Odor-modulated upwind flight of the sphinx moth, *Manduca sexta L. J. Comp. Physiol.* 169: 427–440.

Winkler, I., Kujala, T., Tiitinen, H., Sivonen, P., Alku, P., Lehtokoski, A., Czigler, I., Csepe, V., Ilmoniemi, R. J., and Naatanen, R. (1999). Brain responses reveal the learning of foreign language phonemes. *Psychophysiology.* 36: 638–642.

Wong, C. W. (1997). A brain model with the circuit to convert short-term memory into long-term memory. *Med. Hypotheses.* 48: 221–226.

Yanagisawa, N. (1996). Historical review of research on functions of basal ganglia. *Eur. Neurol.* 36 (suppl 1): 2–8.

Yarbus, A. L. (1967). *Eye Movements and Vision* (translated from Russian by B. Haigh). New York: Plenum Press.

Young, C. M. (1989). Selection of predator-free settlement sites by larval ascidians. *Ophelia* 30: 131–140.

Young, J. Z. (1989). The Bayliss-Starling lecture. Some special senses in the sea. *J. Physiol. (Lond.)* 411: 1–25.

Zadra, A. L., Nielsen, T. A., and Donderi, D. C. (1998). Prevalence of auditory, olfactory, and gustatory experiences in home dreams. *Percept. Mot. Skills.* 87: 819–826.

Zeki, S. (1993). *A Vision of the Brain.* Boston: Blackwell Scientific Publications.

Zhang, S. P., Davis, P. J., Bandler, R., and Carrive, P. (1994). Brain stem integration of vocalization: Role of the midbrain periaqueductal gray. *J. Neurophysiol.* 72: 1337–1356.

Index

as quantifiable, 215–218
as single-cell property, 213–214

Rapid eye movement (REM) sleep, 129–130
Reality. *See* External world
Reciprocal neuronal activity, 6
Reflex activity, 6, 35, 36, 134. *See also* Fixed action patterns (FAPs)
Reflexological view, 42
Refraction, 99
Regenerative firing, 46
Remembering, 185, 188–191. *See also* Memory(ies)
Remote sensing, 98
Repetition, 174–175, 198, 199. *See also* Practice
Representations, 108–109. *See also* Abstraction
Resonance, electrical, 12
Resting cell, 85
Retina, 70, 96, 103
Rhinencephalon, 165
Rhythmicity, coherence, 10, 12
Rhythmic movement and motricity, 48, 203–204

Scallop eye, 101, 103, 104
Sea anemone, 80
Sea animals, 101, 103. *See also specific animals*
Sea squirts, 15–17, 78
"Self," 8, 12, 23
concept of, 127–128, 247
knowledge of, 267
thalamocortical system and the generation of, 124, 126
Self-activating system, 57
Self-awareness, 23
Self-image/self-representation, 226, 247–248, 265
Self-referential behavior, 42, 43, 227
Self-stimulation, uncontrolled, 259, 260

Sensations, as intrinsic events, 156–161
Senses. *See also specific senses*
extension of, by means of spoken language, 248–249
restraining properties, 135–136
secondary qualities of, as inventions/constructs, 128
Sensorimotor images, 1–3, 54–56
defined, 1
Sensorimotor transformation(s), 65–66, 80
Sensory cells, 11
specialization, 80
Sensory cues, 8
Sensory experience(s), 202
center point for, 216, 218
learning, memory, and, 180, 190–192
Sensory feedback, 37
Sensory input, 7
Sensory organs, invention of, 93–96
Sensory pathways, 161
Sensory representation, 114–117
Sepia, 240, 263
Sessile, 15. *See also* Sea squirts
"Shadow," 174–175, 199
Sharks, 59–60
Simplification of reality, 108
Simultaneity, 67, 121–123
Single-cell motricity, embedded to form a system, 58–59
Single-cell organisms, 75, 113, 213
Single cells, 213, 219
as giving rise to single models, 69–72
use of intracellular and extracellular "tools," 76–78
Skin, receptors in, 111, 112
Sleep, 208. *See also* Dreaming and wakefulness
REM, 129–130
Song of birds, generation of, 138–141